PRAISE FOR *THE SPEL*

"*The Spellers Guidebook* is one of the most important entries into our libraries of parent advice books today. When we 'assume competence,' support and break down motor planning, and work with fine motor deficits, including visual motor skills, we can tap into the gifts and emotions of our nonspeakers. If you know anyone whose verbal communication skills are unreliable, limited, or nonexistent, this book is the key to unlocking their thoughts, feelings, and more. Thank you, DM and Dana, for helping us understand that 'not speaking' does not mean 'not competent.' "

—**Patricia S. Lemer, MEd, LPC, author of *Outsmarting Autism*, director emeritus of Epidemic Answers**

"*The Spellers Guidebook* is required reading for anyone who is curious about the Spellers Method of communication for nonspeakers. This book provides a comprehensive, yet user-friendly overview of how to get started on your own nonspeaker's spelling journey. Dr. Dana Johnson and Dawnmarie Gaivin have done an excellent job describing the basis for and the logistics of this new, groundbreaking modality that provides robust communication for all autistic children and adults who are nonspeakers or unreliable speakers."

—**Brian Hooker, PhD, chief scientific officer of Children's Health Defense and father of speller Steven Hooker**

"This is the miracle manual for which the parents of nonspeaking children have long been waiting. If you've tried everything and feel hopeless, rouse yourself one final time to read this fantastic book and take action to help your child break through years of silence. My daughter was twenty-three years old when she made her breakthrough. The first session she was melting down and I had Dawnmarie ask her, 'Do you have faith that this can work?' With a shaking finger, she spelled her first word. 'NO.' Three months later, I had Dawnmarie ask my daughter the same question and she spelled 'ABSOLUTELY.' Our non-speaking children are desperate to communicate with the world and show their intelligence. I believe this program can work for any child."

—Kent Heckenlively, JD, *New York Times* **bestselling author**

"This guide is a must-read for families seeking communication and hope for their nonspeaking loved one. Having once taken communication for granted, I can't convey how hard it has been to accept the news that our daughter may never speak. However, after reading this book and working with the Spellers team on motor and regulation preparation for her to spell, Spellers has become our path for unlocking limitless opportunities and capabilities for our young daughter."

—Meg Gill, entrepreneur and cofounder of Golden Road Brewery; named *Forbes* **30 under 30 (2014)**

"Spelling as a path to communication is life-changing and transformative in the lives of nonspeakers and their loved ones. When my son, Nicholas, who has autism and limited/sometimes unreliable speaking skills, developed the ability to communicate through a letterboard, he spelled out, 'Spelling has freed me from my silent prison.' That's when I understood the depth of my son's thoughts and capabilities that I had been unaware were trapped inside him. For new and seasoned parents, this *Spellers Guidebook* is the perfect companion to take along the journey with your loved one who is learning this method of communication. You'll undoubtedly have questions as you move forward, and all are well answered in these pages. I am excited for all readers because I know that the possibilities are endless of what spelling can unleash for others like my son."

—Jacqueline Laurita, TV personality and mother to speller Nicholas

THE
SPELLERS
GUIDEBOOK

PRACTICAL ADVICE FOR PARENTS AND STUDENTS

DAWNMARIE GAIVIN
AND
DANA JOHNSON

FOREWORD BY J. B. HANDLEY

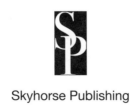

Skyhorse Publishing

Skyhorse Publishing books may be purchased in bulk at special discounts for sales promotion, corporate gifts, fund-raising, or educational purposes. Special editions can also be created to specifications. For details, contact the Special Sales Department, Skyhorse Publishing, 307 West 36th Street, 11th Floor, New York, NY 10018 or info@skyhorsepublishing.com

Skyhorse® and Skyhorse Publishing® are registered trademarks of Skyhorse Publishing, Inc.®, a Delaware corporation.

Visit our website at www.skyhorsepublishing.com.
Please follow our publisher Tony Lyons on Instagram @tonylyonsisuncertain

10 9 8 7 6 5 4 3 2 1

Library of Congress Cataloging-in-Publication Data is available on file.

Hardcover ISBN: 978-1-5107-7969-3
eBook ISBN: 978-1-5107-7970-9

Cover design by Brian Peterson

Printed in the United States of America

Contents

Foreword

If you are the parent, loved one, or caregiver of a nonspeaker or unreliable speaker, you've come to the right place.

The life of my family and our son Jamie can be clearly delineated into two parts: life before spelling, and life after spelling. Life before spelling was frustrating, scary, anxious, and unknown. Life after spelling? Glorious, hopeful, exciting, and clear.

I'm not kidding. Jamie, our beautiful son who was diagnosed with autism at eighteen months old, just turned twenty-one. For seventeen of his years, Jamie was a nonspeaker with no means to communicate. As he aged, he became more frustrated. As he aged, my wife and I became more fearful on what the future held, both for him and for us.

·And then on a beautiful day in January 2020 in Oceanside, California, we met Dawnmarie Gaivin, hereafter in this book known as "DM." In our case, due to lots of hard work and plenty of luck, Jamie was spelling open sentences in no time.

For those new to spelling, the word "open" needs to be explained, because it's mind blowing if you've spent a decade or more raising a nonspeaker. "Open" means a nonspeaker can use a letterboard or keyboard to spell original thoughts and words. I'll give you an example, this from a recent conversation that Jamie had with DM (we still go to Oceanside monthly to practice spelling), DM asked the question, Jamie spelled the answer:

Q: What does nostalgia mean?

A: It's not feeling sad about the past but feeling reminiscent in a good way.

Q: Use the word plethora in a sentence.

A: I'm so lucky to have a plethora of good friends to celebrate my birthday with this year.

Q: How would people describe your personality?

A: My boyish charm is balanced out by my bold determination.

I have several thousand more examples of interactions like these, but I think you get the point. These are the words of a young man who was relegated to a life skills class, who experts informed us had a deficient intellect, and who society had largely given up on.

The two amazing women who wrote this book have never given up on our kids. I already told you about DM. Her coauthor, Dana Johnson, has also been an integral member of the team that has brought Jamie to where he is today. Not only did Dana further Jamie's spelling skills when we paid her a visit at her clinic in Tampa, but her emphasis on integrating his body movements and building his initiation skills have greatly improved Jamie's autonomy and independence. We were able to do this through dozens of zoom calls with Dana.

I'm not an OT, SLP, BCBA or any of the other myriad service providers who work with our kids, I'm just a dad. The only thing that has mattered to me or my wife Lisa is Jamie's quality of life and quality of experience. Four years ago, before spelling, we were imagining a quiet life for Jamie on a farm somewhere, in nature, hopefully surrounded by other nonspeakers, and giving him the richest life we could. This plan was complicated by the fact that we had no real idea of what Jamie wanted, and he had no way to tell us.

Today, our plans are clear. Jamie is presently finishing online, neurotypical high school. He wants to go to a great college, with his spelling friends. After that he'd like to be a neuroscientist. Life after spelling is good. Enjoy the ride and never give up. They can all do this.

J. B. Handley
Portland, OR
August 22, 2023

Introduction

WHAT IS SPELLING?

The word *spelling*, as defined by the Oxford Dictionary, is the process of writing or naming the letters of a word. Anyone capable of reading this page already knows that letters are joined together in a variety of combinations to spell unique words, and those words are considered single "units" of language. When language is shared from one person to another, that is how communication happens. The definition of communication, therefore, is simply the exchanging of ideas or information between two or more people.

All pretty straightforward, right?

Except in the world of nonspeakers, not quite.

Spelling, as the term is used in the world of nonspeakers and minimal speakers, is far more than just a simple term or idea. It is literally *life-saving medicine,* as described by Evan Tastor, nonspeaking cast member of the award-winning documentary film *SPELLERS.* Spelling as a form of communication is the means by which thousands and soon millions of people are being freed from their lives of silence. Spelling in this context isn't simply a descriptive term explaining how letters become words. Spelling means access. Spelling means autonomy. Spelling means liberation. Spelling means everything!

BULLET POINTS

If you're the *CliffsNotes* kind of reader, here's a quickstart version of this handbook. On one page, it's all the steps you need to take to get started teaching spelling as a form of communication to your nonspeaking loved one. Additional details on these items are found in the pages that follow:

Step One: Learn all you can about these three technical concepts:

   a. Praxis—a.k.a. motor planning
   b. Apraxia—difficulty with motor planning, and the fact that it's consistently inconsistent
   c. The difference between measuring someone's *motor* skills versus their *cognitive* skills, and how that has been the great misunderstanding of nonspeakers and minimal speakers all this time.

Step Two: Learn how to presume competence.

Step Three: Find a practitioner who will do (at least) your initial assessment for you *in person*.

Step Four: If you can't get an appointment quickly with a local provider, read the rest of this handbook and consider signing up for the next Spellers online communication partner training course, offered every nine weeks. There you will be assigned an experienced practitioner who can work with you remotely for eight weeks. Visit www.spellers .com/crp-online-training for next start date.

Step Five: Buy stencils and lessons for your home sessions (visit the Spellers store for both or www.SpellersLearn.com for more lessons.)

Step Six: *Practice . . . Practice . . . Practice.* Daily spelling sessions of at least fifteen to thirty minutes is ideal.

———————————————

FROM THE AUTHORS

Dawnmarie (DM)

As I sit here reflecting, it's as if I spent the first forty-five years of my life on a wild bronco that was taking me on its personal joy ride through the wilderness. I'd often grip the reins and try to steer it back in another direction—gosh, any direction would be better!—but it would quickly humble me back into acceptance of my powerlessness. Though the scenery was often beautiful, I wondered many nights, "What is the point of all the miles I'm traveling?!" Then one day, it became crystal clear. In 2017, through a series of serendipitous events (which now happen *all the time*), I embarked on my professional journey to teach spelling and typing to nonspeakers. I quickly discovered that the wild bronco beneath me had been training me the whole time. Among many other useful life hacks, it taught me to trust my intuition, be confident in my values, walk the fine line between pausing and taking bold action, and leap into the unknown with reckless abandon when a situation calls for confident leadership.

My beautiful sons, Evan and Trey, are the muses who thoroughly groomed me for this new life of service. They taught me how to love unconditionally, give without expecting anything in return (ever), have gratitude for the little things, and be patient with myself and others. Today I don't hold the reins of life so tightly anymore because clearly everything works out exactly how it's supposed to. By honoring my values and myself, I was privileged to be part of the incredible documentary *Spellers*; I've been blessed with the world's greatest work partner in my ride-or-die, Dana Johnson; I have the most compassionate and dedicated staff at Spellers Center-San Diego; and I get to spell and type with nonspeakers in our Ohana every single day. If I'm dreaming, I hope I never wake up because life can't get much sweeter than this.

There are millions of people to thank, but I'll sum it up with just two gamechangers. J. B. Handley, thank you for absolutely everything. You are one of the most generous and bighearted humans alive. You are always being of service to other autistic children and their families!

I feel so lucky that the stars aligned, crossed our paths, and made us friends. And to my mom, Pauline Gaivin, thanks for showing me what resiliency looks like. If it weren't for your example, I know I would have been thrown off the horseback in the bucking bronco years. Everything I've been able to accomplish points directly back to you and your influence on my life.

For everyone who bought this book because you're embarking on your child's spelling journey, welcome! I'm so happy to have been given the opportunity to cocreate this handbook for you. Hopefully, you find answers to your questions along with the inspiration to stick through the initial learning process. It won't be easy sometimes, but I promise it will all be worth it!

In gratitude,
Dawnmarie

Dana

Full disclosure—sitting down to coauthor a book was admittedly not something that was on my list of things I wanted to accomplish as a professional. Mainly because I don't feel that I am a good writer. I have difficulty putting my thoughts on paper. I loved my clinical work as a PhD student but struggled to finish my dissertation. I can talk all day long but writing content is very challenging. However, when I look back on my life it was always the times that I chose to "jump into the uncomfortable" that really changed me not only as a person but also as a professional. Writing this book was definitely one of those times. Over the years of learning about apraxia, the brain-body disconnect, spelling, nonspeakers, and unreliable speakers, essentially all the things I didn't learn in OT school, I knew I needed to put what I had learned into a handbook of sorts so that other professionals and parents could learn what I had learned. I had been asked multiple times by parents, "Is there a book that I could read that talks about everything you just said?" I would always laugh it off and say something like, "No, but I should really write one!"

This book was long overdue but was written at the perfect time. It's been a labor of love and many times I have stopped to really appreciate that I get to do what I do every day. I am so thankful to Dawnmarie who texted me one day and asked if I had a moment to talk. I quickly replied "Yes" and called her. She asked me if I would consider hosting a week-long "family camp" for spellers and their families so they could start spelling sooner with their child because waiting lists were long. Another risk but I didn't think twice. "YES!" I replied. And here we are but I couldn't do this without the support of my team at Spellers Center-Tampa. Thank you for showing up each day with the same passion that I have. To the person that keeps the clinic open and my life together, Taryn. You are the only one that can put up with me. It's probably because you have had forty-one years of practice!

There are many that have supported me in this journey, but I am most grateful to my husband, Todd, who has been so patient with me and all of my crazy ideas. I love you more than you know! To all the nonspeakers whom I have worked with—you have changed me. I am not the same person that stepped out of grad school. I have learned and will continue to learn from you. Thank you for allowing me the privilege of working with you and your family. I don't take one moment of it for granted and I am committed to providing reliable communication to all 31 million nonspeakers worldwide.

Finally, to all those who have purchased the book, thank you! You may be a parent, caregiver, clinician, or just interested in learning more. To the parents, I am thrilled that you are starting your journey to hear your child's voice for the first time. Even though I may not ever meet you, I am just as excited for you as I would be if you were stepping into my clinic for the first time. To the clinicians reading this book, I am excited for you too! Spelling changed my perspective as a clinician and my hope is that it changes yours as well. Now, let the revolution begin!

Dana

1

Spelling for Communication

If you're a nonspeaker, which means you're a person who can't use speech as your most reliable and effective method of communication, how *do* you share *your* ideas? Well, let's assume you don't have autism or apraxia but instead someone put tape over your mouth therefore you're unable to speak. How would you communicate? You might write your thoughts down and email or text them. You might gesture, use sign language, or make facial expressions to represent your feelings. You would probably get really creative and find as many ways as possible to express yourself to the people around you, especially those you love the most.

But what happens in the case of someone who has limited or poor motor control, such as after a stroke or ALS? This is where communication gets a little more complicated. In this population of people who become nonspeakers, most had been speech users before the onset of their medical condition. This single fact—as in the case of Stephen Hawking—means everyone around them presumes they're still intelligent even though they no longer use their voice, tongue, articulators, etc., to communicate. Stephen was still seen as a thinking, feeling, and frankly—brilliant—human being. His lack of speech was viewed entirely as a motor disability. Though I cannot imagine how difficult it is to lose your ability to speak, nonspeakers who fall into this category are less marginalized than the next group of nonspeakers we will discuss.

So yes, let's talk about the autistic and Down syndrome nonspeakers. Or those born with cerebral palsy or other conditions which may result in little to no speech. The educational and medical community often presumes incompetence or a lack of intelligence for children who fall into these diagnostic categories. For decades it has been believed that a nonspeaking person is also nonthinking. Because of their lack of effective communication, they are often spoken to and taught like small children long into their teenage and adult lives. Happily, in recent years that storyline has begun to change, but it's still the default mindset in many communities.

So why do assumedly well-meaning educators, physicians, and therapists often presume a lack of intelligence in our kids? Historically speaking, when given an IQ test, most nonspeakers score in the lowest percentiles. When given novel one or two-step directions and zero coaching, many nonspeakers cannot comply or do so incorrectly. Through these informal tests and other standardized assessments, students with little or no speech are often diagnosed as having language deficits, language processing disorders, or as intellectually disabled. They don't "pass" the tests. But like any good researcher, it's always best practice to analyze whether your study design measures what you think you're measuring or whether a potentially confounding variable is at play. In the case of nonspeakers, evidence has been mounting for years that points to the latter being true. That unaddressed variable is called apraxia.

Apraxia, dyspraxia, developmental coordination disorder, sensory-motor processing disorder, sensory integration disorder—the issue that impacts a nonspeaker's ability to pass tests and prove their intelligence goes by many names. SLPs, OTs, and teachers might argue the definitional nuances, but they all boil down to difficulty with "praxis" or intentional movement. These conditions involve the complete inability to do something—such as speak—or the failure to do something on demand and accurately. The intensity of apraxia varies from person to person and often results in students having splintered skills. For example, we've seen students who've mastered particular motor skills thanks to high motivation and years of practice but can't do the same thing *on demand* to achieve another goal. One example we often hear is, "but my son can already type!" Upon further inquiry, we find out they can type their favorite YouTube video titles into the Google search bar, a skill they painstakingly taught themselves to do years earlier. Now it's an automatic, memorized muscle sequence they can do like wildfire. But they cannot type to answer questions or have conversations (yet). Welcome to the world of apraxia. It's consistently inconsistent.

But guess what? There's great news—we can help!

Disclaimer: There are many existing methods that teach communication through assistive technology such as letterboards and keyboards. This book is meant to be descriptive only of the Spellers Method. Though the authors are previously trained in S2C (Spelling to Communicate), this is not an official handbook of S2C or any other method other than Spellers Method. If you are working with a provider of any other spelled or typed communication method, please refer to that provider and their authorized resources for specific training in their methodology. For more information on Spellers Method please, visit www.spellers.com. Thank you and best of luck to you on your journey ahead!

IDENTITY-FIRST/PERSON-FIRST LANGUAGE

Throughout this book, you will find a variety of terms used to describe our clients as well as their communication partners and caregivers. We'd like to take a moment here to acknowledge that the speaking autistic population vastly prefers identity-first language. This means referring to someone as "autistic" instead of describing them as a "person with autism."

Until spelling methods became prolific and nonspeakers began to develop the ability to self-advocate, parents and educators turned exclusively to speaking autistics for guidance. Who better to give us insight into what *might be* the lived experience of a nonspeaker than a fellow autistic person? But today we have thousands of nonspeakers who can fluently type and spell to communicate for themselves. They now have the agency to explain to their teachers and loved ones how they identify and which terminology feels most affirming to them. In our Spellers Centers, as soon as clients become fluent, we ask these exact questions. We have found—initially to our surprise—that many of them do *not* identify as autistic at all! We've also found that even more prefer person-first language over identity-first language. The word choice preference is apparently as diverse as the autism spectrum itself.

Since this book's primary purpose is to support all families and new spellers on their quest to communicate, we are attempting to appeal to the aggregate. We will alternate our use of person-first language with identity-first language and ask for grace from our readership if this is a particularly sensitive topic for you. Consistent with how we treat our clients—each one as a unique individual with preferences, needs, and sensory-motor profiles—we honor their right to describe themselves with the words of their choosing.

We always welcome feedback and suggestions from the neuro-divergent community. Their lived experience is the most important part of any method or movement designed to support them; after all, "nothing about us without us" is a foundational principle of the Spellers movement.

WHOM DOES SPELLERS METHOD HELP?

An understandable first question! Over the years everyone has heard of some therapy or intervention that "miraculously" helped somebody else's child, but how do you know if it will help yours? In the case of Spellers Method your child will benefit if they are a:

- Nonspeaker
- Minimal speaker
- Unreliable speaker (someone who scripts, is echolalic, can speak but cannot answer questions reliably, and/or cannot have a conversation)

Essentially, if speech is not an effective method of communication for your child then using some form of spelling or typing, guided by a trained practitioner, will likely help.

The second most common question we are asked is, what age is a good age to start? Followed by, is there an upper limit? Meaning, does this not work if begun after a certain age? Generally speaking, a student as young as four or five years old is often ready to begin this process although students start at any age. Contact a practitioner to discuss your child's unique profile to help decide if it's the right time for you!

Also, it is *never* too late to start spelling. Currently in our Spellers Center, the oldest client we have is fifty-eight and she is achieving the same success as the younger students! Her now elderly parents are excitedly learning to become communication partners as well! It's quite a beautiful sight.

A detrimental concept that once permeated the autism service industry was the idea that there's a limited "window of time" to positively impact a young autistic person's development. Furthermore, if a child wasn't communicating by age eight then they had little hope of doing so. This just isn't true. Thanks to neuroscience and the concept of neuroplasticity, we know that the brain can adapt, create new synaptic connections, and improve functionality at any age. In the world of spelled communication, we have seen this happening for years. We haven't needed MRIs to validate what we see transpire in front of our eyes time and again after months of steady practice on the letterboards. Student after student, the evidence has shown us that the brain is capable of making new neural pathways and the resulting motor skill output improves. This byproduct of neuroplasticity is open communication in nonspeakers long past eight years old.

HOW DOES SPELLERS METHOD WORK?

Let's get right to the heart of it. How exactly does spelling on a letterboard turn into a form of reliable communication for nonspeakers?

By lowering the amount of neurological effort required in the brain (in the motor cortex, to be specific) to initiate and execute sequences of planned muscle movements, students previously thought to be intellectually disabled have an easier time following directions. To say it even simpler, in Spellers Method, we start by making the targets we're asking a child to point to much larger (i.e., each letter is three inches tall), and we hold the alphabet board up vertically to ease the demand on the eyes (controlled by fine motor muscles). Doing so has significantly reduced the amount of motor planning required. Since fine motor muscles require more brain power than gross muscles, we try to avoid as many fine motor muscles as possible (such as the muscles involved in speech) and use the speller's shoulder and arm instead to reach for the target letter. When they hinge forward from the shoulder and poke a letter on a vertical letterboard with a pencil, the motor planning, or praxis, gets easier.

Then, we coach the child to coordinate their eyes and hands to move together towards the correct target. We do this by verbally prompting the child until they master the skill. They practice, practice, practice, and we coach, coach, coach. Over time, the student learns to correctly select letters in sequence and starts to spell words independently. But before students can use a letterboard for communication, they must develop a sustainable rhythm and accuracy on the boards. This requires several steps and is best done with a trained practitioner to achieve the smoothest path to fluency. Guidance from a trained practitioner is also critical to avoid possible influence. If a speller isn't accurate but is trying to converse with you on a letterboard, you are walking on very thin ice together. The communication will likely break down, and the chances of you misinterpreting their intended message are high. Good practice is critical to avoid such hazards.

In a nutshell, that is how spelling methods work. Step one is finding a local practitioner or someone to consult with over Zoom for coaching and guidance. Step two is lowering the motor demand. Step three is prompting and coaching the student to execute the motor movements successfully. Step four is to strap your seatbelt on as you quickly approach a future full of new possibilities for your nonspeaker!

WHAT IF MY CHILD CAN'T SPELL YET?

This is a common question and misconception. People often mistakenly believe that their child cannot spell or read because their child can't demonstrate otherwise! Dawnmarie made this erroneous assumption too about her own son, Evan.

Currently all tests used to measure reading or spelling ability are based on motor tasks, making it difficult for nonspeakers with apraxia to show the full extent of their intellect. Your child has been listening and learning their entire lives, even though their body has been telling you otherwise. To reassure you further, every nonspeaker who's become fluent has shared (when asked) that they could read and spell at a very young age even though they couldn't demonstrate it by pointing to the correct letters.

We promise that your nonspeaking child is no different. They understand more than their motor skills have been able to show. They do not need to prove they can spell before starting this method.

WHAT IF MY CHILD IS INTELLECTUALLY DISABLED (ID)?

The premise that motor planning differences could be at the root of nonspeakers' communication difficulties is just beginning to be acknowledged; however, the research supporting that claim has been accruing for some time. When taught the motor skills needed to organize their body's gross motor movements, move their eyes, coordinate looking with pointing to a target correctly, children diagnosed with autism, Down syndrome, cerebral palsy, alleged intellectual disability, and other conditions *can* and *do* show their intelligence.

In all formal assessments and informal trials done of nonspeakers, there is no accommodation made for their motor planning difficulties. To pass such tests, students must be first taught the motor skills required to show their knowledge. Otherwise, how can they show what they know? Only *after* being given a reliable communication method can an educator, therapist, or medical provider accurately assess a child's cognitive abilities. I'll say that again. Only *after* being given a reliable communication method can an educator, therapist, or medical provider accurately assess a child's cognitive abilities. Assessing a nonspeaker without teaching them the motor skills needed to take the test, is the same as judging how smart a fish is by whether it can climb a tree or not.

If your child has been given an ID diagnosis or some other label implying profound cognitive impairment, believe they *can learn* the motor skills to correctly identify letters. That's all you have to believe to start this journey of spelled communication. *If they've ever learned to do anything themselves*—shut a door, bring you your keys when they want to go somewhere, put a shirt on—*they can learn motor skills*. They can learn this too. Finding letters with your vision and touching them with your finger or a pencil is a motor skill. Presuming competence starts by believing they *can learn* to do this. You don't have to believe anything yet about how smart they might truly be under the heavy cloak of apraxia.

Culturally, when facing a decision, we often ask ourselves, "What do I stand to lose if I try this?" Instead, we ask you to consider asking yourself, "What do I stand to gain?" Imagine those possibilities and welcome to this next chapter of your life!

2

For the Agnostics Out There

We understand that by now, as parents and caregivers you've acquired a stack of reports from very reputable and well-meaning professionals that say your child has a cognitive disability, or at the very least, a receptive language delay or processing delay. You can probably also tell a host of personal stories that seem to validate those official assessments. So why should you jump on this proverbial hope train and believe that everyone before must have been wrong? Why should you believe the various spelling method practitioners (*who must have ulterior motives, right? After all, they get paid to teach this stuff!*) who are telling you to presume competence and to believe that your child can already spell? And what about that one agency with an actual position statement stating this method and other forms of letterboard communication have been "debunked?" Why would they say that if it could truly help the 31 million nonspeakers out there? It just doesn't make sense.

Words from DM: We get it. I get it. I have to admit, it has always perplexed me that just about every touchpoint in my boys' autism diagnosis, treatment, and education has been layered in either controversy or red tape. Nothing has ever been simple or straightforward. Why does the world seem to make our parenting decisions so hard? It's not like autism parenting came with a handbook. For goodness sake, every parent I know is doing the best they can based on the information they have and their personal beliefs. If only people "out there" could trust *us* and support *us* while we make our own educated decisions on behalf of our child. Just like they do for parents of neurotypical children.

So, speaking of beliefs, if you've seen the movie *Spellers* then you may remember the moment in my interview when I described myself sitting in the rocking chair of my younger son's nursery. In that rocking chair, I contemplated life now that both of my sons had autism. Whether it was due to a scarcity mindset or simple practicality, I believed I had better prioritize my long-term goals for them because there would never be enough of me or enough resources to do it all. There was no question in my mind that robust communication was my number one goal for them both. I knew communication would help them be respected, stay safe, and create meaningful relationships. If they each could attain those three things then I would be quietly satisfied with my life as their mother.

By the time I was ready to give letterboards a try, I had done everything else. All day, every day, I was modeling communication. We had mastered PECS, we had trialed other forms of low-tech AAC, Evan was rocking a speech generating device for requesting, and he had developed a small repertoire of gestures paired with vocalizations that our family understood. But his communication was far from robust. He had proven, however, that he was fully capable of learning despite what the standardized tests tried to tell me in his IEP meetings. Going purely on my belief that he could learn anything if taught with patience and perseverance, I told my speech language pathologist my plan.

"You know what *'they'* say about those methods, right?" she asked.

"Yeah, I've done my research. They say that the instructor is the one influencing the student's output," I replied.

"Yep. So they say," she answered.

I looked at her and shrugged, "Except that *I'm* going to be his instructor. I'm going to have the RPM teacher show *me* how to do it, and then I'm going to teach him. Why on earth would I influence my own son's communication when the whole point of me doing this is so I can get to know him better?"

She smiled at me and replied, "I totally agree and think you should go for it!!"

And the rest, as they say, is history.

The point of sharing the above story is simply to say that, like DM, you are in charge of this journey with your child. If you believe that your child has ever learned something before, believe they can learn this. If you believe in neuroplasticity, then you already know a little bit about how the brain can rewire. If you believe that paradigm shifting ideas have always caused a bit of an uproar before things settle down into a new understanding, then you might not be surprised that there are critics to these methods. You might also remember the words of Schopenhauer:

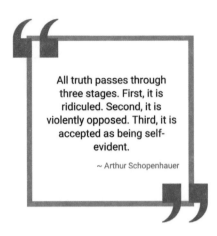

> All truth passes through three stages. First, it is ridiculed. Second, it is violently opposed. Third, it is accepted as being self-evident.
>
> ~ Arthur Schopenhauer

Once you see your own child spell out their thoughts and ideas, you can't unsee it. The truth becomes self-evident.

Watching your child become a *Speller* is a paradigm shifting process for everyone whether you'd been completely on the fence or were ready to jump in with both feet as soon as the first session began. We promise, you don't have to shave your head, change your name, or drink any Kool-Aid to embark on this journey. You just have to open your heart to the possibility that you too might experience the life-changing moment of hearing your child's first true words, spelled on a letterboard.

3

Reasons You (Might) Think You Can't Do This

Though we cannot possibly list all the reasons someone might hesitate to start their Spellers Method journey, we came up with a few common things we've heard.

1. You don't have the money.
2. You don't have enough time.
3. You have other kids/competing priorities.
4. You're afraid that it won't work.
5. You have a (secret) fear that it will work.

Though neither of us were business majors, we're going to present you with a little cost benefit analysis before specifically responding to the above legitimate concerns.

Who doesn't like dessert first? So let's start with the benefits! What do you stand to gain from teaching your child to spell for communication?

1. The end of ambiguity. No more guessing what they specifically mean when they say "bah" and make a new gesture with their hands that you can't figure out. No more wondering what hurts when clearly they're sick and something is wrong. No more worrying that they cannot tell you what happened when they aren't with you. What an incredible concept—soon you can just ask them on their letterboard and they can tell you this information firsthand.

2. You will finally get to know your child, and we mean: the *real* <insert your child's name here>. For years you assumed that the things they gravitated towards repeatedly were preferences, whether those things were certain colored shirts, certain video characters, or certain music. But now you can find out why and if those really were preferences or simply motor habits (which we sometimes call "loops"). Getting to know your child's thoughts, feelings, passions, dreams, and ambitions are even more rewarding and these become accessible through spelling as well.

3. Let the carpool lane conversations begin! No more zoning out in the car on drives with your nonspeaker. Now you know to capitalize on a great opportunity to fill their brain with juicy podcasts, informative news stations, and other audible material for discussion once you're parked and can pull out a letterboard together. Knowing now that 100 percent of what you've been saying all these years has been understood by your child now means that every minute you're together is an opportunity to share that moment in a deeper way than you previously thought. How amazing is that?

4. Now you get to help your child overcome the public perception that they weren't intelligent or that they

REASONS YOU (MIGHT) THINK YOU CAN'T DO THIS

had nothing to contribute to society. Although the world at large is still pretty heavily laden in ableism, as the army of spellers grows and this civil rights movement rolls forward on behalf of nonspeakers around the world, they simply cannot be ignored. And with this rise in awareness and call for social justice, your child will lean on you as an ally and advocate for them, just like always, only now they will be self-advocating through their spelled communication as well. What a powerful team you will make together!

5. The number one thing a parent of a child with autism worries about is "What will happen to my nonspeaking child after I'm gone?" Although most of our nonspeakers still have high support needs due to their motor planning challenges, the sheer power of them having a reliable form of communication alleviates one big worry about the future. A world full of possibilities opens up once someone can communicate with the people around them. More employment opportunities, more relationships, more educational access, more of everything! To know that your child will be able to express themselves fluently to future caregivers means they will be understood and their needs will be adequately expressed by them. You won't need to be there to speak on their behalf.

Ok, so we've taken care of the benefits. Now what is it going to cost you? This brings us to the list we made previously of common objections we hear.

1. You don't have the money. Philosophically speaking, what price is too high to hear your child's authentic voice? But practically speaking, know that you don't

have to work with a practitioner weekly in order to successfully learn this.

Dawnmarie only worked with a trained practitioner on three separate weekends over an eighteen-month period. Besides that, she did all the rest of her son's coaching herself. Like DM, you do not need to break the bank on this modality. Also, depending on where you live, you often can use regional center or state waiver funds for these services but you'll need to coordinate with your local spelling provider to make those arrangements. Last but definitely not least, there are nonprofit organizations with scholarship programs available to get you started if money is an obstacle. SpellersFreedomFoundation.org is dedicated to this cause and others have created programs to support nonspeakers access to reliable communication.

2. You don't have the time. Believe us when we say, we know that time is everyone's most precious resource. Although best practice is spelling daily with your nonspeaker at home, they will still make steady progress if you spell with them three times a week for twenty to thirty minutes each time. Even better is if you can spell five times a week for fifteen to twenty minutes a day. The point is, consistent shorter practice is better than sporadic marathon long sessions. We would also like to offer you the idea that if you make connecting with your child the primary objective of your spelling session rather than accomplishing spelling (see the chapter on coregulation for more details on this) those fifteen to twenty minutes will be the highlight of your day.

3. You've got other children or competing priorities for your attention. This one can be tricky to navigate without a doubt and the best thing we can say is that life certainly isn't fair. Yes, your other children may sacrifice a bit during the acquisition phase of your speller's journey, but the payoff to the family as a whole will be massive once fluency is achieved. If you consider your family like an ecosystem, a change in one part of the system always affects the rest of the system. A positive change in the life of their sibling will benefit them dramatically as well. Depending on the ages of the siblings you can certainly involve them in the spelling practice or lesson prep, and of course seek family counseling to navigate the unique needs that pop up for your family members. Stress is stress, even when it's exciting, positive, and life-changing in all the right ways. Siblings and you may need a little extra support handling the stress even though it's for a good cause.

4. You're worried it won't work. We've all chased that elusive white rabbit one time or another, and now we're just "over it." You've done everything, tried everything, and are too tired to embark on something new. Rather than be redundant here and repeat the last two sections (which you might just want to reread) we'd highly recommend you talk with other spelling parents. You're sure to find many parents who were also hesitant or skeptical at first and they can share their wisdom with you. At the end of the day, however, we think the least dangerous assumption is to give spelling a chance rather than resist it due to contempt prior to investigation.

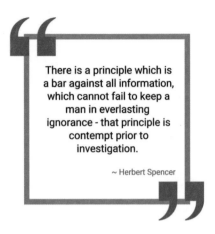

> There is a principle which is a bar against all information, which cannot fail to keep a man in everlasting ignorance - that principle is contempt prior to investigation.
>
> ~ Herbert Spencer

5. Maybe you're worried that this method *will* work, and you find yourself reading this book riddled with guilt about things you've said in front of your child in the past. Or perhaps you're ashamed about how you treated them before you realized they were always listening and understanding. First of all, you are not alone. Many parents have done the things you've done, thought the very same thoughts and felt the same feelings. If it's any comfort to you—and we do hope this is comforting— rarely if ever does a new speller speak out negatively against their parent or caregiver. Typically, they are so overjoyed at their communication liberation and they are grateful for you bringing this method into their lives that the past is forgiven on the spot.

6. If you do find yourself experiencing a lot of mental anguish around such memories, we highly recommend you seek out a family therapist to process these feelings with. Doing so will ultimately help support your journey as a communication partner with your speller. Clearing out the old history along with feelings of guilt or shame from your heart will put you in a much better position to serve as a communication partner.

Have we convinced you yet that the cost-benefit analysis leans more in the direction of this being beneficial? We hope so. But you do your own calculations as well as soul-searching and recognizance. There is no urgency on our part to get you in the spelling saddle, though your nonspeaker might have a different vote.

YOU'RE STILL AGNOSTIC, BUT YOU'VE SCHEDULED AN ASSESSMENT!

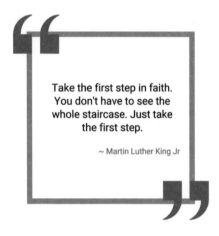

> Take the first step in faith.
> You don't have to see the
> whole staircase. Just take
> the first step.
>
> ~ Martin Luther King Jr

Okay, so you've taken the first step and made an appointment . . . congratulations! This decision likely brings both excitement and anxiety as you anticipate the possibilities. As parents of children with minimal or no effective speech, you have become master sleuths at interpreting their attempts to communicate. Without a doubt, you're more than ready to stop the guessing. You've got millions of other questions for them too, along with a deep longing to know them in a more intimate way. What do they think about? What do they yearn for? Do they really still love Elmo or are they stuck in loops watching the furry little red monster? How do they feel? Do they have dreams for the future? All of the possibilities swirl through your head and the adrenaline starts to kick in. Your heartbeat quickens and maybe you hold your breath. At that moment, for some of you, the amygdala in your brain sends out an alarm. "Hold on, just a minute! Let's shut down this daydreaming nonsense *just in case.*" In submission to safer ground, your thoughts turn to: What if *my* child is the one this won't work for? We have chased many elusive white rabbits. What if this becomes another huge waste of time, money, and hope? What if the professionals who told me this is a debunked methodology are right?

But . . . what if, as J. B. Handley states in the award-winning movie *Spellers*, what if they are *wrong*? Which of these is the *least dangerous assumption*?

As their parent, you've always suspected that your child understands everything and is capable of more. Maybe you've seen inconsistent skills—one day they can follow two-step directions perfectly and the next day they can't seem to identify a familiar object you named. Even though deep inside you haven't fully believed the professionals in your life, you have come to terms with the idea that your child probably has a cognitive disability since they can't prove otherwise. To now sit on the precipice of learning a new method of communication, one that would defy all the prior "evidence" of your nonspeaking child's cognitive disability, can be a scary thought. It might bring regret over the lost years when you trusted the therapists, educators, and other professionals who said your child is only capable of certain things. Or it might bring fear that you won't be enough for them. That you're too tired, too old, or not smart enough to do this yourself. Have no fear. We are here to assure you that you've made the right decision!

We understand and applaud your brave step forward. As Martin Luther King stated, you don't have to see the whole staircase to take that first step.

You are *not* alone on this journey. Practitioners are trained to support you in the skill acquisition phase for both you and your speller (yes, start calling them a speller!). Meanwhile, other parents, caregivers, and CPs are here to support you through the emotional ups and downs. You can connect to them on our Facebook group, Spellers Community, which is open to all. It is moderated specifically by practitioners trained in Spellers Method, but the community goes beyond methodologies. The time has come for spellers, allies, and advocates to work together so nonspeakers can achieve their rightful place in society. Community connection is essential to share resources and build resilience in ourselves and our nonspeakers.

One last word (for now) on all the "evidence" that therapists and professionals told you meant your child wasn't intelligent. As a person with apraxia, your child has difficulty with their body's intentionality and putting their thoughts into action. They do not have an inability to learn and understand. They have an inability to move their body purposefully to prove they have learned and do understand. As soon as they learn the needed motor skills, you get to find out who they really are!

BUT MY CHILD CAN "TALK"

This may be one of the biggest roadblocks for some to start spelling. We put so much emphasis on speech in our world that parents of unreliable speakers may not know how Spellers Method might be appropriate for their child. We work with many unreliable speakers who have shown tremendous success with spelling. Unreliable speakers are those that have speech; however, what they say is not necessarily what they want to say. Many unreliable speakers have verbal "loops" or words/phrases that they say repeatedly. For example, they may walk into a restaurant or store and say things like "Time to go home" or "All done"; however, that often isn't intentional. Our spellers with unreliable speech have told us on their letterboards that often what comes out of their mouths is not what they really wanted to say. Some even tell us not to respond to their speech because that makes them more frustrated. This can, of course, be very confusing especially during academic testing when their cognitive ability is assessed using their speech output. They typically test below grade level and are then given academic work that is below their true ability.

Unreliable speech tends to come in phrases that have been practiced or repeated over and over again. What happens when we practice a motor movement repeatedly? It becomes automatic and permanent. Unfortunately, when the same phrase is repeated, even when it's not in the appropriate context, parents may think it is intentional. Most often the unreliable speaker does want to say something; however, the connection between their expressive language center and their articulators is disrupted. This leads to some over practiced phrase or verbal loop to come out instead.

Many of us want our children to speak and when they do, we want them to continue to practice speaking. Unfortunately, and unknowingly, we might be hardwiring phrases or words that then become loops. We will talk more specifically about motor loops later in the handbook. For now, just know that if you're the parent of an unreliable speaker, spelling is a way to ensure they have a means to reliably communicate. By bypassing the fine motor skills needed to speak, your child can communicate more reliably. If left exclusively to their own speech, you might only ever know the tip of the iceberg of their true thoughts and feelings. With spelling, you'll find that they not only have the ability to have a full conversation but their vernacular is often very different from what comes out in their speech. It's more robust, more mature, and more detailed.

This is why we encourage parents to start spelling even if their child has speech! In the film *Spellers*, Madison is one of the unreliable speakers who found a new freedom through spelling her true thoughts. What she could say verbally was far less than her incredible intellect was thinking. Through spelling and now typing, she's attending college with her typical peers.

BUT MY CHILD IS TOO "COMPLICATED"

Every speller has a different sensory-motor profile. Some are not bothered by loud noises or intense auditory stimulation, yet others are highly sensitive. Some spellers have more complicated bodies and may be unable to extend their arm or isolate their index finger to point. For still others, it might be incredibly challenging to get their head and eyes to look forward, let alone maintain their gaze on the letterboard. Some spellers may have limited mobility, have a low vision diagnosis, are in a wheelchair, or are unable to sit in a chair. Guess what? They all can spell, too! Yes, they may take longer to build the motor skills required to point to the letterboard and coordinate their body movements, but they can do this!

We work with many families who hesitate to start spelling because their son or daughter may have a genetic abnormality, a more complex motor diagnosis like cerebral palsy, or multiple diagnoses in addition to autism. All of these families have been able to work on spelling and have built the motor skills needed to reach a letterboard with twenty-six letters. One caveat is that these families all work regularly with a highly-trained practitioner. Most of these families also work with an occupational therapist who understands the interplay between apraxia and spelling. Lastly, many of them also work with a developmental optometrist so that any ocular motor and vision needs are considered. As a result of this interdisciplinary approach to spelled communication, the needed modifications to the letterboard itself, board placement, and access points are incorporated. Some spellers may need the letterboard to be in a different place or the size of the letters to be smaller or larger. Your Spellers Method team will be able to individualize spelling to what your child's unique sensory-motor profile needs for successful spelling.

Your child's sensory-motor profile may include self-injurious behaviors or injurious toward others. You may be too worried that your child may hurt themselves or the practitioner, so you avoid trying this. We want future spellers to feel their best, so if any medical issues need resolution, we highly suggest they be addressed first. However, some spellers have experienced past trauma or are highly anxious, resulting in the dysregulation of the body and the challenging behaviors we see. Spellers Method practitioners are trained to support the speller, help them regulate, and brainstorm with you about their individualized needs. The goal of the spelling session may not always be to spell. With more complex motor profiles, the goal might be to regulate, to get their eyes on the letterboard, or to isolate the index finger.

Ultimately, we don't want your child's more complex body to deter you from scheduling your first session. If you're unsure, set up a time to talk with the practitioner so that your questions can be answered. It's important that you understand the process, but it's even more important that your child has a voice!

4

Things You Can Do Right Now

Prior to heading to your first session, we recommend that you and your speller check out a few resources:

- Watch the film *Spellers* (www.spellersthemovie.com /watch). This 2023 documentary film takes a look at the lives of eight nonspeakers who spell or type to communicate. It provides a glimpse into the real-life journeys of the families and how each nonspeaker was introduced to spelling.
- Read the book *Underestimated*—written by Jamie Handley, a nonspeaker and typer, along with his dad, J. B., about their personal journey and the highs and lows they experienced as a family. It was when they found spelling that everything changed. The film *Spellers* is loosely based on the book.

- Read other books written by spellers and typers. A full book list can be found in the bibliograph.
- Talk with other parents of spellers. If you don't know any, join our Spellers Community Facebook group or feel free to reach out to us through www.spellers.com. We are always happy to put you in touch with other families. Community is one of the most important things that we value. Connected families are strong in their support network and a great way to learn from each other.
- Learn all that you can about apraxia and the brain-body disconnect. Our spellers struggle to put their ideas and thoughts into action. They do not have a cognitive disability but rather a motor planning disability. This is a *big* mind shift for most families and reading up to learn more about not only the challenges but how you can support them to gain control of their bodies will help your whole family.
- Google what books or literature are age appropriate for your nonspeaker and try reading a little to them out loud each evening. Don't ask them to read the text themselves, even though they can. At this point, you do the motor work. Some students need to practice handling the sensory input of a person's voice reading so don't worry if the sessions are short at first. Just start the routine. And as long as they are in the room with you and not watching an iPhone or iPad movie, it counts. Listening doesn't have a "look" so trust they are hearing what you're saying.
- Begin to presume competence. As we have mentioned earlier, we must fully presume competence in our nonspeakers. But what does that mean exactly? And is it an instantaneous thing like a "burning bush" moment, or is it a gradual process? The answer to the latter is—it can be either, but regardless of how quickly it happens, it's foun-

dational to successfully teaching spelled communication methods. Presuming competence means that you believe your child understands you and has the ability to learn age-appropriate concepts. Because of this, it is important that you talk with your child about the first session. Tell them what you have learned by reading this book and through talking to the practitioner. This will help them know what will happen at the first session. This is such a foundational concept to Spellers Method that we have another chapter dedicated to it further along in the book.

5

Preparing for Your First Session

"SHOULD WE BRING REINFORCERS?"

A frequently asked question from new spelling families is whether or not to bring reinforcers to the assessment session. Typically, this question is asked by families who use applied behavioral analysis (ABA) services either at home or school, and they've found that snacks or treats encourage their child to participate longer in less preferred or more challenging activities. We have good news for you. We'd actually prefer that you do *not* use reinforcement during spelling sessions. Here's why . . .

We would like you and your child to be open to having a whole new experience! After all, this will be the first day of their whole new life as a speller. That means it's time to set aside everything you think you know about their motivation to work, their interest in learning new things, what their "behaviors" mean, and especially about whether they're smart enough to understand why they're doing this. *Spoiler alert: they* are *smart enough!* We want to give you the opportunity to see things differently. To see how "top-down" regulation can be just as effective as "bottom-up" (see "Top-Down versus Bottom-Up Regulation" on page 120 for further explanation).

When given the just right challenge along with the appropriate level of motor coaching and support, the need for tangible reinforcers becomes nil. We frequently have school districts or private Board Certified Behavior Analysts (BCBAs) come to observe spelling sessions with students and they sit in awe of how the student can sit at the table and spell for forty-five minutes without any reinforcers or breaks. Meanwhile this same exact student at school requires reinforcement every five minutes to stay "on task."

If you start out by using reinforcers during spelling sessions on day one, when would you fade them? *How* would you fade them? Your child would be expecting them and they'd become part of the routine. As a result, you'd never get to see this inspiring ability they have to sustain attention and work hard simply for the chance to master something with pride! We want to give you the opportunity to presume a whole new level of competence in your child. But don't worry, you don't have to know how this is all going to work. You just have to trust us that it's possible and let us show you the way.

Meanwhile, the other reasons we avoid reinforcers is because we'd like to model alternative ways of regulating your child. We'd also like to show you how we coach their bodies rather than give verbal "first-then" contingencies. Our goal is not compliance. Our goal is coregulation. Remember, communication is ultimately their choice. We don't want to force it on them. We want to woo them to work hard despite their apraxic bodies and to believe in themselves again. Many students come to us with a very fixed mindset about their abilities to do anything successfully if it requires intentional movement. They have spent years trying to successfully point to a flash card on demand, or arrange letter tiles to prove they can spell, all with little success. Many have simply given up trying. We are here to show them they *can* do this and we will *help* them be successful. By doing everything differently—no reinforcers, coaching motor not cognitive, using top-down regulation techniques along with bottom-up, they can have a whole new experience of themselves as a student. It is a whole new design for learning that you're about to embark upon.

THE NEED FOR AMPLE REST

It's difficult to say this without imagining most parents rolling their eyes, but try to have your speller get a good night's sleep. Especially if your child has a seizure disorder, we cannot overemphasize the importance of this. If you're traveling to see a practitioner, we would even suggest adding an extra one to three days on the front end so you can settle into your normal bedtime routine as much as possible. Simply put, your child is about to do a lot of work. Plan to get as much rest as possible. In other words, don't overdo it when you come to town even if the greatest theme park on earth is just a few zip codes away!

COMPLETE THE INTAKE PACKET

Please be sure to complete and return the intake questionnaire sent to you by your spelling practitioner at least a week before. Please don't hold back from being honest regarding your child's behavioral history. It's important for us to know what is possible and if there are triggers we should be aware of. We cannot prevent all dysregulation but we like to be prepared and curate the environment as best we can. After all, without regulation it's difficult for your nonspeaker to learn anything. The body's nervous system can't be in fight or flight mode and a social/engaged mode simultaneously. Working together as a team we will do our best to create a space that feels safe and supportive to you and your child.

DON'T PANIC IF THE FIRST SESSION IS BUMPY

Many, if not most, first sessions go off without a hitch! But if one session is going to be particularly challenging it's usually the first. The biggest reason is because all of this is new for every single family member involved. Caregivers might feel anxious because they aren't sure their speller will be able to do it. Thoughts and doubts might creep in along with anxiety about whether their child will be regulated or not. From the speller's perspective, the clinic may be a brand-new space for them to visit and they've probably never met the practitioner prior. They may have heard about spelling on a letter-board from their caregiver, but aren't sure what's about to happen. Performance anxiety can make their first session more dysregulating. Yes, ripping off the proverbial Band-Aid of that first session can be anxiety-provoking for everyone, but that's 100 percent okay! Emotions are high with excitement and anticipation.

When emotions are elevated, that can bring dysregulation and impulsivity to an all-time high. Practitioners expect that the family will be nervous and new spellers are going to be more dysregulated, so please don't worry about it! We are experienced in this process and can't wait for your speller to get started.

NO TIME FOR CHIT-CHAT UPON ARRIVAL

When you first arrive, you will notice a few things that are different right from the start. First, we speak directly to the speller even though they may not be able to respond. We know they understand and we want to help regulate and make them (and you!) feel comfortable. The practitioner will introduce themselves to the whole family and then bring everyone into the room where we will jump into spelling immediately. We will explain the process to the speller while the caregivers observe and learn. We do ask that caregivers hold their questions until the latter part of the session so that we can get into flow with the speller. This helps to reduce the anticipation and heightened emotions that they might be experiencing. As we get the speller on the boards and we begin to teach the motor skills needed, their brain and body get more connected and everyone will slowly become more comfortable.

As practitioners we know that each speller's sensory and motor profile will be different. Some spellers will experience more impulsivity and dysregulation. This may cause the speller to be self-injurious or injurious toward others. We completely understand this and place no judgment on the speller or the caregivers. In fact, our main goal at that point would be to help the speller to regulate their body, but oftentimes we will also continue to spell. Experienced practitioners are familiar with dysregulation and know that it can be difficult for everyone. We will work through it and talk through it with you.

WHO SITS WHERE?

We not only welcome parents into the spelling sessions, we require it! So please plan to sit in and learn alongside your speller. We don't recommend a giant audience in the room though, so if you've brought your extended family with you it might be best to choose two, maybe three, people to come in. You will sit in the available chairs along the back wall of the room while your speller and the practitioner will sit in front of you, but facing a table. (In other words, you're looking at their backs, but you can still see the spelling happening.)

The speller will sit on the left-hand side of the practitioner. Seating is an important aspect of successful spelling and the practitioner may change the chair to ensure that the speller is supported to sit upright, not slouching or leaning to one side. Observing the speller's posture is important. Core stability and postural control can affect the accuracy, endurance, and stamina of the speller. The practitioner will make adjustments as necessary.

LESSON STRUCTURE

As the practitioner starts to read a short paragraph from a pre-written lesson, you will notice that they've chosen an age-appropriate topic for the speller. Although you might be worried because your child has never been exposed to this level of content before, rest assured, they are soaking it all in! We presume competence and that starts even before they've demonstrated their knowledge. We will continue to present this level of material to them because we know this also helps to regulate them. In the chapter on regulation we will discuss further how age-appropriate, high-level content supports the regulation of the speller. It's a strategy called "top-down regulation."

Next the practitioner grabs a letterboard. We always start with the lowest motor demand. That means we use the three letterboards during our assessment lesson even if the speller has some prior experience with another practitioner. Seeing the basic motor planning required on the three boards gives the practitioner information that guides the rest of their clinical judgments.

Next, we practice the motor skill of holding the pencil with the appropriate grip. If we feel that the speller cannot maintain the proper pencil grip or simply won't use it, we might try using a high contrast sensory foam board instead. When using these letterboards the speller can poke the letters with their finger instead. Our gold standard, however, is to use the three stencil boards and a pencil whenever possible. This ensures that the speller really hinges from the shoulder and pokes cleanly in and out of each letter.

Next, we practice the motor skills of finding and poking the letter on the stencil board. This often isn't as easy as it looks for the speller. For some, the "simple" movement of poking a letter is very challenging. It requires a tremendous amount of body coordination and for someone with apraxia, this is very complex. The practitioner will continue to read about a topic from a lesson and the speller will continue to practice poking the correct letters. As the session unfolds, you will notice that your speller often needs some guidance or prompting to get to the right letter. This isn't "cheating" or "dumbing it down." We are helping them to build the motor planning skills needed to do it on their own. Remember, we aren't testing their cognitive abilities. At this stage, we are simply teaching them the intentional motor skills to scan, find a letter, and poke it.

Think about when you learned a new motor skill—playing an instrument, learning a new sport, or another skill. You probably hired a teacher or a coach. If you're more the self-study kind of person, you watched multiple YouTube videos in order to learn the steps involved. The same is true for your speller. They need a "coach" to help them learn the steps involved in this motor skill. The practitioner is their new coach who will help them through the process of scanning the board with their eyes and accurately selecting the target letter(s).

While coaching, the practitioner will also be assessing. They will take careful note of how the speller's body is coordinating its movements. For example, do they look for the letter, then poke? Do they look for the letter, look away, then poke? This provides us with a lot of information on how the speller's eyes and body work together. Many spellers have difficulties with their eyes. A frequent difficulty we see is with fixation or the ability to hold the gaze on an object (i.e., keeping their vision on the letter they intend to poke). Another common challenge involves eye teaming or the ability for the brain to use the eyes together effectively. Additionally, any deficit in actual visual acuity will also affect spelling and could make things very difficult, possibly resulting in dysregulation. Rest assured, the practitioner is trained to assess for motor differences in the area of ocular motor and can make the proper referral for you to a developmental optometrist as needed. We talk more about vision in the chapter on sensory-motor differences.

WHEN YOU CAN'T BELIEVE THE ACADEMIC LEVEL BEING PRESENTED

You may observe your speller working with the practitioner and wonder "Isn't the content being read to my child at a level that is too high academically and cognitively? My speller has not been exposed to these words or this type of material. How are they understanding all of this?" Great question!

Let's talk about the difference between speech and language. Speech is purely a motor task. Moving your articulators, the fancy name for the muscles that move your lips, tongue, and jaw, in order to produce speech sounds is a highly coordinated fine motor skill. Language, on the other hand, does not require moving muscles. We use our cognition to create ideas, to think about our response to someone's question, or to comprehend a lesson you might be listening to. Since these language-based activities occur in the language centers of the brain, they do not require the muscles of your mouth to get involved. At least, not until you want to say out loud the things you've been thinking, understanding, or deciding. So, these two processes— speech and language—are actually two separate tasks, although as mentioned, they do work together when someone speaks in order to share their ideas. It is erroneous to assume that absence of speech means absence of understanding or intellect.

Our spellers have motor planning difficulties because of what is called apraxia. We will get into the specifics of apraxia in a future chapter (or you can jump ahead now), but simply stated apraxia prevents the speller from putting many of their ideas into action. There is a breakdown in the connection between their brain and their body. The speller might have an idea but isn't able to get their body to initiate and get the task done. This may be new information to you so take a few moments to really soak that in. It is also challenging to understand when your speller is consistently inconsistent with their motor skills. Sometimes they can do a task, sometimes they can't. But with apraxia, your speller's ability to complete motor actions on demand may be compromised even though they understand what you are saying or what you are asking them to do. The cognitive part, that is, wanting to answer or to do something, does not simply make the motor part "go."

This concept of apraxia is not new, even though you may not have heard of it before. Apraxia and other related motor planning differences have been studied for a number of years by researchers including Dr. Elizabeth Torres. Her research focuses on the disruptions in the sensory-motor feedback loop affecting the intentional movement of the individual. More on this later. Let's get back to the first spelling session.

ADJUSTING TO YOUR SPELLER'S UNIQUE SENSORY PROFILE

As the spelling session unfolds, something will be happening that you may or may not have picked up on from the start, and that is how the practitioner supports the speller's regulation. Each speller has an individual sensory-motor profile and some may need more regulation support while others need less. Practitioners will adjust the volume and speed of their voice, use a more "singsong" tone to help get into a rhythm, or even suggest the speller engage in some breathing exercises to help reduce the sympathetic nervous system activation and support overall regulation. The tools we employ to maintain the optimal level of arousal are endless, and knowing your speller's sensory-motor profile is essential in the CP and speller relationship.

Board choice, seating accommodations, insertion of intentional motor exercises before or during the lesson, various tools to poke letters with . . . the adjustments made by the practitioner throughout the first lesson are endless and are all in response to their assessment of your child's sensory-motor profile. Our goal is to make these clinical decisions for you and set you up for success from the start. Because your child is a human organism who is constantly changing and growing, these initial decisions can and do evolve over time. That's the main reason we recommend families get guidance here and there from a trained practitioner. Part of our job is to think three steps ahead and prevent any bad habits from starting in the first place, rather than try to break motor loops that might occur when the wrong tools or techniques have been employed.

IN SUMMARY

The practitioner's goals for the first session are:

- First and foremost, to establish a trusting relationship with the speller and their family. Spellers have come from all different experiences. We want to ensure that everyone feels comfortable and supported by the practitioner.

- Observe and take mental notes of the speller's sensory-motor profile. Specifically related to:
  - Ocular motor skills
  - Gross motor skills
  - Stamina and endurance
  - Overall regulation
- Determine which letterboards are best for the speller to begin with based on the above assessment and determine if any modifications are needed. It may take a couple of sessions before a final decision is made, but most of the time it can be ascertained in the first evaluation. Our gold standard is to start every student we can with the three stencil boards with a pencil/stylus. This combination helps to really teach the speller to hinge their forward movement at the shoulder. That said, if the student's eyes or motor profile need a different board, that's okay. We will select the board that will reduce the motor demand most effectively to allow for smoother acquisition phase progress. This is where the guidance of a trained practitioner is so critical to getting off on the right foot.
- Build your understanding of the difference between motor and cognitive.
- Build your child's confidence that they *can* do this.

6

What *to* Do, What *Not* to Do

Most, if not all, parents want their children to be successful. Parents of nonspeakers are no exception. When the opportunity comes up for their child to work with a practitioner to learn the motor skills to spell, parents and caregivers *really* want their child to be successful. As practitioners, we want that too but it's important to remember that learning the Spellers Method is just like learning any new motor skill. Both the child *and* their caregiver are brand-new to the method, so learning from a trained practitioner is the best way to go.

For the most successful session for your child, here are some pointers:

- Do be honest with triggers and repertoire of injurious behaviors before coming in. As mentioned earlier, the intake packet sent to you by your practitioner is not trying to weed you out based on your answers. The questionnaire is designed so we can prepare for your child's session thoroughly. When we know as much as possible about a speller, we can support both the speller and caregiver to be successful when spelling.

- Don't talk about your child in front of them as if they aren't there. It might be an old habit—we get it—but practice speaking about them the way you would a neurotypical child who would be standing there. Remember, we presume competence so using the term "potty" for anyone over the age of four isn't presuming competence, and when we don't presume competence, we aren't showing respect to our spellers. We know it's a process and we will encourage you to shift your vocabulary so it becomes a habit.

- Try to just watch and let the practitioner coach your child during the session. We know this can be *really* difficult to do especially because your child is going to miss-poke and make mistakes when they are spelling. It can be difficult to see and may even cause you to doubt your child's ability but let us take the lead and feel free to ask questions or offer to help *after* the practitioner is finished and there is an opportunity for questions.

- Do offer to help if your child's dysregulation becomes injurious especially if your child is bigger than your provider! This is a tough one because dysregulation and impulsivity are triggered by emotions and sensory overload. During the initial spelling sessions, emotions run high for both the child and the caregiver. The speller can often pick up on their caregiver's emotions which adds to the possibility of impulsivity and injurious dysregulation. It's natural for feelings of excitement and anxiety to occur, especially in the first few sessions. As the expert on your child, if you know the signs of dysregulation or when there may be injurious dysregulation, please let us know beforehand so we can be prepared and perhaps take a break before anything happens. If you offer to help and the practitioner says, "Don't worry—I've got this," trust them and let them handle the dysregulation. (We know how hard this is!)

- Don't coach your child from the back of the room; let the practitioner run the session and be the one coaching your child to poke the correct letters. Yes, it's human instinct to want to help your child either not feel anxious or to perform really well. Learning a new motor skill is difficult but part of our assessment is to watch the pattern your child pokes with and what aspects prove to be difficult for them. We can then individualize what your child needs based on their unique profile. You've always been your child's biggest cheerleader and advocate. They know this, and we know this! But now's the time to sit back and (silently) cheer them on while you watch.

- Try to pay attention to what the practitioner is doing, not just your child. Of course, during the very first session your eyes will be mostly on your child because you can't wait to see how they respond. But eventually, you'll be the one learning to be a communication partner, so it's important to watch the practitioner too. Most practitioners videotape their sessions for you to watch back later, so that's helpful. We highly recommend watching the recordings so you can learn to mimic the practitioner's board placement, verbal coaching, and coregulation strategies.

- And last but not least, breathe. Don't forget to breathe!

7

Clinical Concepts to Understand

Most, if not all autism parents are familiar with certain clinical terms and may very well be sick of hearing your child described using these words. Our goal here is to simply ensure that you have an understanding of what your child may be experiencing. Learning these terms is an important part of fully understanding your child and their individual profile.

PRAXIS

The process of intentionally moving our bodies is called praxis. In occupational therapy (OT) terms we call it executing a motor skill. By definition, it's our ability to put our ideas and thoughts into action. There are a number of steps involved in the process of praxis and these include:

1. Having an idea
2. Planning, sequencing, and organizing that idea

3. Initiating the movement to start acting upon the idea
4. Executing the movement(s) to complete the idea
5. Adjusting the body should something "go wrong"
6. Inhibiting the body once the idea is completed

Example:

1. Idea: I'm thirsty.
2. Planning: I know there's sparkling water in the fridge. I'll go get some of that.
3. Initiating: the body starts engaging muscles to pause the TV and get up off the couch.
4. Executing: I begin to make all the muscle movements needed to walk into the kitchen, reach for and open the fridge door, visually scan and find the water, reach for the bottle, pull it out, shut the door, twist the cap off, and lift the bottle to my lips, purse our lips, tip the bottle, and swallow the water as it enters my mouth.
5. Adjust: If I reach into the fridge and grab the wrong bottle I have to adjust and look again, find the correct item, and grab that. Or if I can't open the bottle, I have to move my body to find someone or something to help get it open.
6. Inhibit: When I'm done swallowing enough water, I have to lower the bottle from my lips and place it somewhere.

Each of us go through these steps consciously while learning any new motor skill. Here's an example most people can relate to. If you have your driver's license you probably remember the first time you got behind the wheel and how much you had to think in order to move your body through the steps to drive. But once you have practiced a new skill repeatedly, the movements then become more unconscious, or automatic, and you are able to do the task without as much thought. Again, thinking about driving, you've practiced the motor skills of driving a car so frequently that even though you encounter novel traffic patterns every time you get behind the wheel you are able to think about and do other things (talk on the phone, pass out food to back seat passengers, listen to an audiobook) while driving. The praxis required for driving is now automatic.

Now think about the last time you learned a new motor skill—an instrument, sport, or new recipe—you most likely had to put all of your focus and thought into moving your body to complete the task successfully. Now that you have practiced the skill over and over, you don't have to put so much thought into it. That is, unless you unexpectedly hurt your dominant hand making it impossible to use. Once again you have to put more cognitive effort into the task because the automatic motor skills are lost due to the shift in the coordination of the body. It's quickly relearned, however, because we have the ability to quickly build the motor patterns needed for success.

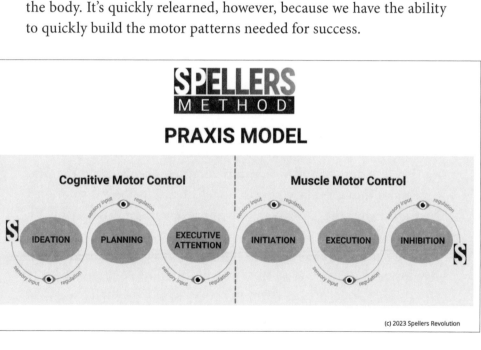

APRAXIA

Apraxia is the breakdown of praxis. It's the condition where an individual can't complete the steps of intentional motor planning due to a neurological difference even though they can understand what is being asked of them. Other terms often used in place of apraxia include: dyspraxia, developmental coordination disorder (DCD), sensory integration disorder, sensory processing disorder, motor planning differences, fine motor delay, gross motor delay, behavioral disorder, and the list goes on. What's important to remember is that apraxia is *not* a cognitive issue. This is true even though many diagnosed with nonspeaking autism have also been the label of cognitive delay or intellectual disability. The "evidence" often used to justify these secondary diagnoses is simply the person's inability to respond accurately to our requests. It is important to know that apraxia described here refers to whole body apraxia. You may have heard the diagnosis "childhood apraxia of speech" or CAS. This is a diagnosis given by speech therapists and refers to an inability to move the articulators (muscles around the mouth to speak) to produce speech. We use the term *apraxia* throughout this book to refer to whole-body apraxia.

Apraxia is prevalent in 67 percent (www.pubmed.ncbi.nlm.nih .gov/26114615/) of those diagnosed with autism, making intentional movement of their body very challenging. What makes things even more difficult is that apraxia is "consistently inconsistent," meaning that one day the individual can complete the task and the next it seems as though they've never done the task before. It's not only frustrating for the caregiver, but it's even more frustrating for the individual.

So, what if everyone was wrong in assuming the individual has a cognitive disability rather than a motor disability? Think about it. All assessments that your child has done in the past have required them to write the answer, say the answer, or point to the answer all of which require intentional movement or the ability to purposefully move the body to answer based on what your brain wants to do. To date there is no assessment that does not involve intentional, purposeful movement. We need to consider the stark reality that none of the cognitive-based assessments your child has done are actually measuring what they are supposed to.

SPEECH VERSUS LANGUAGE

Let's talk about communication. By nature, everyone is to some degree a "multi-modal" communicator. This essentially means, we find a variety of ways to get our thoughts across to others. That said, there *is* one thing in common with every form of communication in order for that exchange of information to occur effectively. Have you guessed it? Yes, it's intentional or purposeful movement.

If we want to email, text, speak, gesture, or even use a facial expression to convey our thoughts or feelings, all of these actions require us to move our body intentionally. Nonspeakers and unreliable speakers with autism have apraxia which makes them inconsistently able to communicate reliably. Words often come out that are not what they intended to say. Or they may point to the square instead of the triangle when asked to identify the correct shape. It can be very confusing when the person knows clearly in their mind what they're trying to say or do, but their body defies them. It's equally perplexing for the rest of us who, prior to this book, have been asking the nonspeaker in their life to demonstrate what they really know by pointing to *this* or doing *that.* The sheer fact remains that until we teach their bodies the *motor skills,* we can't accurately assess their knowledge base. So for now, we operate under the least dangerous assumption. You can read more about that in "Presuming Competence" on page 58.

Intervention for a lack of speech tends to be the primary focus for most parents in the early years of an autism diagnosis, and rightly so. By nature, we are communicative beings and we want to be able to communicate with our children. But what are we talking about (no pun intended!) when we say "speech"? Speech, simply put, is our ability to move the muscles surrounding the mouth, the tongue, and vocal chords to utilize our breath purposefully in order to produce sounds that come together to form words. Speech is a very fine motor, purposeful skill. In fact, it is one of the finest motor movements of our entire body. And, spoiler alert, having speech or not has nothing to do with intelligence.

The cognitive part of communication is what we call language. That's the interpretation and processing of what you hear when another person speaks to you, and it occurs in the language centers of our brain. Speech is the motor skill and language is the cognitive skill. Expressing your ideas and thoughts does depend on motor skills—such as speech—but understanding and learning does not depend on these motor skills being intact. Also, very importantly, the lack of speech in an individual does not indicate a lack of thinking. After all, absence of evidence is not evidence of absence.

The interplay of the language centers in the brain and the motor strip as well as the sensory-motor strip are what create purposeful speech. Wernicke's area is the region of the brain that contains motor neurons involved in the comprehension of speech. First identified in 1874 by German neurologist Carl Wernicke, it's where your brain interprets the sounds that entered your ear. If you hear a car drive by, your Wernicke area comprehends that as the sound of a car motor. If you hear a cat meow, your Wernicke area understands that there must be a feline in the area. If someone speaks to you, your Wernicke area says, "Oh, those sounds are words. I hear someone talking. I understand you!" and language comprehension has occurred.

Next, the neural signal travels down a bundle of fibers called the arcuate fasciculus which connect Wernicke's area to Broca's area, otherwise known as the expressive language center in the brain. Broca's area has a busy role of interacting with sensory information from the temporal cortex while also planning a response to the words you just heard from the person talking to you. Once that is complete and you have your own thought or idea to share in response, it sends the signal to the nearby motor cortex to start the motor output process. At this point in time you have not yet communicated a thing to the person standing next to you; however, your receptive and expressive language centers are completely intact and functioning perfectly well.

For this exact reason, we firmly assert that *nonspeaking does not equal nonthinking or non-understanding*. Spellers can and do understand. They learn without being able to speak. There is no accurate way to measure a person's language ability without them having a reliable motoric way to communicate. So, despite what has been believed about them for decades, nonspeakers rarely have receptive or expressive language delays, but rather, they have expressive speech impairments. This is why they need a form of AAC that lowers the motor demand required for communication. We need to address the motor challenges, not assume (erroneously) there is a cognitive delay.

But let's go back to the brain. Once the signal of "I have something to say!" leaves Broca's area in a non-apraxic person, it's sent to the motor cortex which actually has three parts: the primary motor cortex, premotor cortex, and supplementary motor area. Without getting too deep into the neurological weeds here, the motor cortex is responsible for the purposeful or voluntary movements of the body, including the articulators used for oral speech output. If your brain-body connection is working well, the signal then travels down your brain stem to innervate the muscles that make your lips, jaw, tongue and breathing speak out your thoughts in the form of verbal speech. If you have any degree of apraxia or dyspraxia, however, this pathway either never gets started, gets hijacked midway by overly practiced speech such as scripts, or the sounds cannot come out intelligibly. Welcome to the world of nonspeakers, minimal speakers, and unreliable speakers.

The primary motor cortex is arranged into sections that are responsible for controlling various parts of the body. It is said to contain a "motor map" of the body. If you google the term *cortical homunculus* you will see a graphic representation of the motor cortex and how much of it is dedicated to moving (or sensing) particular body parts. Disproportionately represented are the articulators, eyes, and fingers, which makes sense when you think about how much motor planning is dedicated to moving these fine motor muscles. We have now stumbled upon a big reason we strive to reduce the motor demand in spelling methods. If the communication of a nonspeaker gets stuck or hijacked en route from Broca's area to the motor cortex, or from the motor cortex to successful innervation of the associated muscles to speak, then we need to bypass the brain's need to use so much of the motor cortex. Moving communication into the gross motor of the arm/shoulder and having a speller poke letters on a letterboard is much easier than having them speak or jump straight to two-handed keyboard typing which does require finger isolation.

PRESUMING COMPETENCE

As allies and advocates for nonspeakers, we have a choice to make. Presuming competence about nonspeakers is very simply that—a decision. When we decide to presume competence about someone it means we choose to believe that they have the desire to learn, they can learn, and they are capable of understanding what they are being taught even without evidence. Anne Donnellan, Cheryl Jorgensen, and others have argued that presuming competence is typically the least dangerous assumption in the face of not enough evidence. In 1984 in the journal *Behavioral Disorders*, Donnellan described it this way:

> [T]he criterion of least dangerous assumption holds that in the absence of conclusive data, educational decisions should be based on the assumptions which, if incorrect, will have the least dangerous effect on the likelihood that students will be able to function independently as adults. (p. 142)

So what happens if we make a presumption of competence and it turns out we are wrong? What have we risked? Sure, we might overeducate students who aren't fully comprehending all that we are teaching. Would they be more independent as adults had we educated them less? Probably not. On the other hand, if we make a presumption of incompetence and we're wrong, what do we risk? We risk undereducating intelligent, capable students who might otherwise thrive with proper instruction. We risk limiting their potential as a result of us presuming less of them. Which of these do you feel is more dangerous?

Cheryl Jorgensen, an inclusive educator expanded on this concept of presuming competence. She stated that we typically make judgments based on the individual's ability to communicate or demonstrate in some way their knowledge. This judgment affects every decision that we make. We base our beliefs about their cognitive abilities, their physical abilities, and even their future on what they can demonstrate to us. She discusses the least dangerous assumption and poses that exact question we mentioned above: "What are the possible consequences of believing someone is competent should you be wrong?" We can always go back and reteach or provide the necessary support for their learning. If we choose to presume *incompetence*, the effects may be traumatic.

Neurotypical students are never asked to prove their competence before being given access to instruction. They're never forced to prove they can learn or benefit from teaching before being taught in the first place. Yet our educational system does this to nonspeakers all the time. Children with autism are frequently denied access to mainstream classrooms on the premise that they haven't proven they would benefit from the instruction there, despite the fact that federal law states such a demonstration is not required for students to have access to learning environments alongside their neurotypical peers. But these refusals of less restrictive placement, based upon the lack of presumption of competence, happen all the time.

Well, this is not the case with us. In Spellers Method (as well as other methods of spelled communication) the principle of presuming competence is foundational. If we didn't presume competence right away, we would tragically create a self-fulfilling prophecy. If we silently waited for the student to prove they could spell, they would be stuck in their apraxic bodies unable to initiate the motor movement to do so. Instead, by presuming competence, we teach and support their motor while they learn the muscle movements (this is the acquisition phase) and then as they practice, we begin to fade those prompts out as they become fluent spellers. Without presuming competence, the process would stall before it even started.

Some parents will experience a "burning bush" moment of presuming competence. As soon as they see the child find two or three letters correctly on their own while spelling a word, they're fully convinced that all the "experts" before had been wrong about them. For other parents, presuming competence is more of a gradual process. They also notice all the times their child gets to letters without a gesture or directional prompt, and they can see the gradual improvement in their motor skills, but not until something happens that they really didn't expect do they convert to full believers.

> **Dawnmarie:** For me, I always knew Evan wasn't intellectually disabled, but he was also consistently inconsistent with demonstrating his understanding. One day he could follow two-step instructions perfectly, the next day if I asked him to bring me his shoes, he'd hand me a dog toy. So, when Evan answered the spelling instructor's question "What's another word for God's love?" by spelling the word *benevolent* I nearly fell off my seat. Sure, I had presumed enough competence to bring him to the session in the first place. I knew he was *in there*. But I had no idea how intelligent he was. I simply thought he was more educable than the IEP team had made it sound.

All of this talk about shifting your mindset to one of presuming competence is critically important as you embark on this journey. You don't have to see the whole staircase to take the first step, as MLK says. *But you do need to set aside everything you think you know about your child's intellect and learning abilities so you are open to having a new experience.* Once your child has developed enough motor skills to independently scan for and select letters you will have the evidence that they're cognitively right on par with the rest of the world, if not significantly brighter. But if you don't presume competence and prompt while they're learning it will be a dead-end, self-fulfilling prophecy.

8

Gross Motor versus Fine Motor Skills

As the parent or caregiver to a nonspeaker, I'm sure these terms are not new to you. Simply put, gross motor skills are the large motor movements that our bodies can make. Walking, running, doing a cartwheel, or climbing up a mountain are all considered gross motor skills. Fine motor skills are the smaller and finer motor movements that our bodies make. Typing, writing, knitting, and speaking are all fine motor skills. So why is this important to know? It's important because of how and why we teach the Spellers Method the way we do.

Developmentally, as humans we build our gross motor skills *first* and then we develop our fine motor skills. Infants learn neck control first, followed by trunk support (sitting/balance), before they move on to controlling their shoulders, elbows, wrists, hands, and then finally fingers to pick up small items. Gross motor skills are "easier" (we prefer to say "less demanding") on the brain's motor cortex than fine motor skills are. While trying to help someone with apraxia access communication, we want to make the motor demand as easy as possible since it's *really hard work* to begin with. That means putting as much of the process as possible into the gross motor muscles.

When we teach the Spellers Method, we stick to this idea of using gross motor skills before fine motor. That means we teach spellers to utilize larger motor movements first. Rather than begin with typing—which is a very fine motor skill—we start spellers on letterboards that require less precision and fine motor involvement. That means we start new spellers on a set of three stencils, a.k.a. "the three boards," where the alphabet is split across the three boards so each letter is much bigger in size. Board 1 has A-I, board 2 has J-R, and board 3 has S-Z. The larger targets reduce the ocular motor demand and increase the speller's ease of selecting the correct letter without too many errors. Meanwhile, having the speller hinge from their shoulder to reach and poke is more of a gross motor skill than would be typing and moving their individual fingers to find and select letters.

"BUT MY CHILD CAN ALREADY TYPE TO SEARCH YOUTUBE!"

So often new families report this exact statement and then ask whether that means their child needs to start Spellers Method on the 3 stencils. The answer is typically, yes. The reason is this: Although your child has learned, albeit through repeated practice over months and years, to type their favorite, familiar phrases into YouTube, they've developed an isolated but practical skill. This is not the same skill we are working on to eventually elicit open communication. We know that's confusing, because they are using their fine motor skills to type, but not to type high cognitive output such as novel thoughts, answers to questions, homework assignments, etc. And the truth is, if your child could already use their typing skills to communicate, they would most likely be doing so!

It's very difficult (okay, we'll say it—it's close to impossible) for a new speller to start out on a high motor assistive technology device (e.g., typing on a keyboard) and learn to express high cognitive output (communication, not just nouns or requests) without first laying a solid foundation of praxis on a lower motor demand device. In Spellers Method we've found it is purely through lowering the motor demand and starting out on the stencils that we reduce the amount of work required by the brain's motor cortex enough to allow for more cognitive output as skills progress.

As the speller's motor skills improve with practice, we then shift from the set of three stencils to a letterboard that has all twenty-six of the alphabet letters on it. The letters are smaller once put onto the same stencil, but we do have two overall sizes of the twenty-six stencils to choose from. One we call the "large 26," which is about 12" x 18," and the other is called the "small 26," which is the same size as one of the three boards.

Once the speller has progressed with flow and accuracy on the 26 stencil, we move them to a laminated 8.5 x 11" board. Moving to the laminate board is often a big jump for spellers as it requires a great amount of spatial awareness. This is because they are now using a finger to touch the board instead of a pencil that slides into the stencil, which had provided lots of sensory feedback to the speller. This sensory feedback on the stencil helped the new speller know where their hand is in space. Through practice on the laminate board, the speller continues to build their accuracy and their motor skills become more refined. Finally, the keyboard, held by a communication partner and connected to an iPad and app with voice output technology, is introduced as the next step. The keyboard requires significant fine motor skill ability which is why it is reserved for last.

Each move along progression of board types is discussed further in the entry entitled "Motor Continuum" on page 71. It is really important to note that this is where some spelling methods differ from one another. Though we often use the same technology devices (e.g., laminate boards, keyboards, stencils), we do not apply them in necessarily the same way or sequence. It is also really important to remind new families that this is not a race. Making new neural connections in the brain takes time. Steady progress and consistent practice are the keys to laying a strong foundation of motor skills so that as a student progresses along the motor continuum they don't lose the ability to communicate their more complex thoughts due to the increased demand on their brain's motor strip.

> *Authors' Note:* Autonomous typing, sometimes called independent typing (although the latter term is slightly inaccurate), is one additional stage of motor skill acquisition where the keyboard is placed on a stand or flat on the table. Achieving autonomous typing is frequently an aspiration of new spellers, but even more often it's a primary goal of parents for their children to achieve. We understand from the many conversations we've had with families that the motivation to get to this stage is usually rooted in the hope that it will eliminate the need for a communication or regulation partner. For the speller, it also means greater freedom and self-sufficiency, and to never have to wait for an available CP to express their thoughts, feelings, and wishes. All noble and understandable rationales.
>
> Because this step in the motor continuum is so complex and so individualized, we highly recommend working with a practitioner to master the subtleties of it. For a speller to type without a regulation partner is a challenge in and of itself, plus the speller needs to master other motor skills off the boards such as initiation, inhibition, and self-regulation strategies. It is an achievable goal for many and one that several Spellers Method students have attained, but it requires a considerable amount of time and effort to master. Working with a practitioner is highly advised when you achieve this level of fluency. Also, not rushing through the motor continuum to get to this stage is critical. A very strong foundation of fluency must be built on the laminate board even before progressing to the held keyboard, let alone putting it on a stand on the table.

If you rush to that motor stage, you're likely to end up with the same reduced cognitive output due to the high motor demand. No one wants autonomy if it means the speller is back to simply requesting desired items on the technology device.

A very important fine motor skill that is often overlooked is the fine motor movement of the eyes. Ocular motor movements are literally *the finest* motor movements of the body and require a great amount of control. Apraxia makes precise eye control extremely difficult, especially on demand. While the speller is building a new repertoire of motor skills within their spelling practice, don't forget they are also working on the coordination and control of their eyes. Though we have done everything we can to move communication out of the fine motor muscles and into the gross motor areas, we simply can't avoid the use of the eyes to scan and find the letters.

In order for the speller to accurately poke the letter, the eyes need to find the letter first. Then they need to initiate the motor task of lifting their arm and reaching forward to select the letter with their pencil or finger. The hand-eye coordination required can take a lot of practice and can be extremely fatiguing. This is due to the tiny ocular motor muscles responsible for controlling the eye movements. The ocular motor muscles are almost always the limiting factor when building endurance and stamina while spelling. Research in the area of ocular motor function and autism has repeatedly shown that those with autism demonstrate difficulties with saccadic eye movements, fixation, convergence insufficiency, and smooth pursuits (see the appendix for a partial reference list). With that in mind, we highly recommend spellers have a full developmental vision assessment that includes assessing these areas in addition to the traditional optometry measure of visual acuity. Exercises prescribed by the OD and done in conjunction with spelling practice leads to smoother acquisition phase progress.

PROMPTING AND "PROMPT DEPENDENCY"

The question of whether spellers will become prompt-dependent is one of the most common we receive as practitioners. Yes, we prompt them. Sometimes, especially in the beginning, we need to prompt *a lot*. The reason for prompting is to support the speller while they learn to motor plan and build those new neural pathways we keep talking about. With practice they become proficient and then don't need prompting anymore. But if we didn't prompt them initially, how would they learn to do it?

Think back to the first time you attempted to ride a bicycle as a child. Whoever was coaching you probably provided a lot of verbal prompts:

> *Grab the handlebars!*
> *Don't let go!*
> *Push the pedals with your feet!*
> *Keep going... left foot, right foot!*
> *Watch out for the tree! Turn, turn, turn!*

With all that learning behind you, today you can jump on a bicycle and ride it without any prompting at all. That's because years ago your body went through all the individual steps of praxis to create bike-riding motor plan pathways in your brain. Now you can complete the entire sequence of motions automatically. The same thing applies to spelling. We will absolutely fade the prompts as the speller's motor skills and accuracy improve. Just like learning to ride a bike, eventually the speller won't need the verbal coaching because they will have established praxis for the steps involved.

One reason the belief lingers that nonspeaking autistics become prompt dependent is because many times they've never been coached from the motor perspective of things. Therapists, caregivers, and teachers often rely on verbal prompts that simply repeat the instruction over and over. Some even respond with "Nope, try again" when the nonspeaker attempts an action but doesn't execute correctly. This is ironic because if you hired a trainer to work out in the gym and the trainer told you to do a slow negative squat, it would be difficult to execute if you had never done one before. Furthermore, if you made an attempt and it was incorrect, being told "Nope, try again" without feedback on how to do it differently would be equally unhelpful.

Nonspeakers have spent years experiencing situations like this and they've shown us that telling them what to do without coaching their body is ineffective. What they've desperately been missing is someone coaching their body, or "coaching their motor" as we sometimes say. Everyone needs motor coaching to learn how to do motor tasks.

The bottom line is this: *we don't have prompt-dependent spellers because we prompt their motor, not their cognition.* Coaching cognition in students who already fully understand what you're asking them to do but simply *can't* do it without motor practice, is what makes them prompt-dependent. Those prompts rarely work in an activity that requires intentional movement. Once prompts are motor-based, they become effective. Then motor skills are learned and prompts can be faded.

HOW WE PROMPT

There are a number of ways that we prompt to support the motor planning of spelling. First, we have a prompt to initiate poking the letter. Remember, initiating movement is the most challenging thing for those with apraxia. Using strong initiation prompts such as "Ready, set, go!" or "First letter is . . ." each time you put the letterboard in place helps to support the speller's initiation and get their body moving for practice.

Gestural prompts, which are quick waves of the practitioner's finger or hand, are used specifically for the eyes. While observing the practitioner using gestural prompts, it may look like they're pointing directly at the target letter. Early in the spelling journey, they may need to point to the letter to get the speller's eyes directly on it. If the speller can't get their eyes to look at the letter, poking will be very difficult. As their ocular motor skills improve, the practitioner will slowly fade out the gestural prompts.

Directional prompts (e.g., "Up, up, up," "Go down," "Next door," "One over," etc.) also help direct the body to poke the letter successfully. Remember that the speller is practicing the motor planning steps and learning how to do the skill. We aren't trying to measure their comprehension skills. Once their accuracy improves and the gestural and directional prompts are faded, we can then (and only then) consider assessing comprehension.

It's important to remember that certain prompts are specifically reserved for the acquisition phase of spelling. As the speller is acquiring the motor skills to poke the letters, practitioners will need to use more prompts at first. Gestural prompts and directional prompts are the two prompt types that *must* be eliminated before a speller can spell openly. This is important because we want to avoid any chance of influencing the speller's communication. When you gesture to a particular quadrant of the board or verbally coach them in a direction with a directional prompt, you are 100 percent influencing the speller. If a speller continues to require these two prompts, they are not ready to spell openly and need more practice to build their foundational motor skills. Rushing this process will only increase the risk of influencing.

The remaining prompts include eye prompts and continuation prompts. Eye prompts help the speller get their eyes on the board and move their eyes to find the letter. Saccadic eye movements, or being able to shift your eyes to search for the letter, are very challenging for autistic individuals. Supporting the eyes to get to the board with eye prompts (e.g., "Look for your letter," "Look, look,

look," "Get your eyes on it," "Eyes on the board," etc.) all help coach the eyes to the board.

Continuation prompts are meant to help keep the speller's body moving and to support pacing and rhythm when spelling. Apraxia hijacks the body and makes initiating and controlling movements very difficult. Sometimes the spellers poke too fast or too slow. Practitioners use continuation prompts to help the speller's body to continue to move at a consistent pace. Both eye prompts and continuation prompts can be used during both the acquisition phase and the application phase. These prompts do not risk influencing as they don't indicate the direction the speller should take when spelling. Spellers who type on keyboards often need these prompts because of the fine motor demand of typing.

If we consider everything we have discussed to this point—the process of praxis, apraxia, gross motor, fine motor skills, and ocular motor skills—we quickly realize that spelling for communication isn't simply "pointing to a letter to spell a word." It's a whole new motor plan that takes serious practice to master! Some may take a bit longer to become proficient, especially if they have a more complex motor profile, but they can also build the skills needed to spell on a letterboard with all twenty-six letters. You can spell to communicate anything once you achieve fluency on a 26-letter board!

9

Cognitive versus Motor Continuums

MOTOR CONTINUUM

When we refer to the motor continuum, we are talking about adjusting the motor demand from low to high when spelling. Poking the letters on the letterboard is the motor demand. Starting on the three letterboard stencils is the lowest motor demand, followed by the large 26 stencil, the small 26 stencil, the laminate, and finally, the keyboard. When spellers first get to the keyboard, the CP holds it up the same way they did for all the previous boards in the motor continuum.

With each progressive move along the continuum, the amount of motor work that the speller's eyes must do increases while the sensory feedback from the assistive technology device decreases. For example, poking a stencil with a pencil provides a lot of sensory feedback, which helps the speller be more accurate. Typing directly on a device such as an iPad or an SGD (speech-generating device) with your fingertip gives very little feedback, which makes it more difficult. Typing on an actual keyboard does give more sensory feedback with the "click." Still, it is unforgiving, meaning every miss-poke must be deleted, unlike the previous phases of the motor continuum progression. Besides the increased keystrokes needed for deletes, the keys are significantly smaller than the letters on any of the earlier boards. All you have to do is put one of the three stencil boards next to a keyboard to see the obvious difference in ocular motor demand.

Once fluent on a held keyboard, held up by a communication partner, there is a separate acquisition stage for typers where the keyboard is placed on a stand (nicknamed "the cradle" by Jamie and J. B. Handley), and the speller begins to learn to type autonomously. This final step of autonomous typing is a giant motor leap that deserves a handbook all of its own. It's essential for us to mention that not all spellers choose to make autonomous typing one of their immediate goals. Once fluent, they often have other priorities, such as making friends independently, attaining their high school diploma, going to college, joining clubs and recreational groups, and creating a brand-new life full of communication! They've waited a long time to have the agency to determine their own futures. Although we might be eager as parents or practitioners to have them communicate without a CP, it's important to honor their priorities over ours. We also don't want to inadvertently communicate that everything they just accomplished—getting fluent on a letterboard or keyboard—isn't enough. They achieved open communication when they moved up the cognitive continuum while on a letterboard with all twenty-six letters. At that moment, the doors opened to a future full of self-determination, and we need to remember they waited a long time for that moment. The keyboard and cradle can wait if that's their choice.

Everyone has a unique path, and we honor our spellers' choices. The acquisition phase of autonomous typing is exceptionally rigorous, lasts a lot longer than any of the other motor continuum acquisition phases, and slows down the spelling rate quite a bit. That said, every speller who ultimately becomes an autonomous typer is paving the way for those who might not make it to that level.

COGNITIVE CONTINUUM

The cognitive continuum refers to the questions we ask from our written lessons during our sessions. In the Spellers Method, a pre-written lesson is always used when practicing to ensure consistency with how we scaffold the skill acquisition and help maintain regulation. If we always keep the speller competent by proposing the next "just right" challenge to perform, we can support their regulation. If we jump around in our conversation and the range of difficulty in the type of questions we ask goes from way too easy to way too complex, we are likely to trigger anxiety and jeopardize the trust that is building between the speller and the CP.

Lessons are also essential to help the CP stay regulated. If you have to think of a question on the fly or talk about a topic spontaneously at the moment, it can be challenging to keep the flow and conversation going. If you pause to come up with a question, anxiety may start to spike in you, increasing the possibility that your speller will also become dysregulated (see the chapter on regulation for more info). While coaching you to become a CP, we want you to be as regulated as possible. This includes using a pre-written lesson, writing down the keywords as you read, writing questions on a transcript, and recording your speller's answers. It all has a purpose: to support the regulation of both you and your speller.

Here is a sample paragraph from a lesson written by Dawnmarie. You'll note that some words are capitalized. These are what we call keywords. They are typically some of the words we plan to ask the student to spell back, or they are the answers to future questions. While reading this paragraph aloud, you would stop once you read the name Hawking and spell it out letter by letter on the keyword sheet: "H-A-W-K-I-N-G," then continue reading aloud until you get to the next keyword.

> Yesterday morning (March 14, 2018), Stephen **HAWKING** died peacefully at home in Cambridge at the age of 76. He leaves behind an **UNPARALLELED** body of work in

*the world of **PHYSICS** & **COSMOLOGY** (the science of the origin of the Universe) along with an inspiring legacy of how to live a full life while facing intense physical challenges. Diagnosed at age 21 with a rare motor **NEURON** disease known as **ALS** (amyotrophic lateral sclerosis), Professor Hawking was told he had just a few years to live. But the disease progressed more slowly than anticipated! This allowed Professor Hawking to fulfill his destiny as one of the greatest scientists ever.*

After reading the first paragraph, you will see a list of questions below it. The types of questions within the lesson vary. Like the motor continuum, the cognitive continuum speaks to the cognitive demand of the question. The lowest cognitive demand is spelling words. This is where you say "Spell unparalleled" and put down the letterboard with the "U" on it to start the process.

Spell: UNPARALLELED   PHYSICS NEURON

The next move up the cognitive continuum is "known" questions. The term itself means the question has one possible *known* answer. The reason that known questions are higher in cognitive demand is that now an extra step is involved. Before the student can begin spelling their answer, they need to recall or remember the content and retrieve that answer from their memory. Then they must identify the first letter of the answer in their mind and begin the motor execution of finding and poking the letters.

Sticking with spelling words and known questions when a speller is new is essential because you must know what they're trying to spell to coach their motor. Also, when using the three boards, it's impossible to ask them an open-ended question. If you ask a speller, "What do you want for breakfast?" and hold up the A-I stencil, how would they respond if they wanted waffles or pancakes?

Here are some examples of known questions from the Stephen Hawking paragraph above:

(Known)Whoarewetalkingabouttoday?StephenHawking
(Known) How old was Hawking when he was diagnosed with ALS? 21

The next step up the cognitive continuum is semi-open questions, often denoted in the color orange. These questions have more than one answer but typically a finite number of choices. At this point in the acquisition phase, the questions should continue from the content you read in the prewritten lesson. The cognitive motor demand required at this stage is higher now because the speller must recall the information from the passage, think about the answer choices they heard, pick one of those choices, then think of the first letter in that word, then begin the motor process of scanning for the letter and start poking to spell it out. Your speller needs to be on the 26 stencil for most semi-open questions because they need access to the entire alphabet to spell any of the choices. Here is one example from the excerpt above:

(Semi-open) Name one of the two fields of study Hawking contributed to in his lifetime. Physics / Cosmology

Further up the cognitive continuum, we find questions that are either mathematical computations (colored in purple) or previous knowledge-based (colored in blue). Each of these question types increases the cognitive demand needed when practicing the motor skills to spell.

Many parts of the brain are involved in mathematical processing. Signals are sent between the left and right hemispheres' frontal, parietal, occipital, and temporal lobes. Though we begin introducing the number stencil right from the first lesson, we generally only use it to give answers that are quantities or dates. In other words, they are number-based "known" questions. Saving the mathematical questions for when accuracy on the number board is solid allows for no ambiguity on whether the speller miss-poked or miscalculated.

> (Math) How many years did Hawking live with ALS?
> $76-21 = 55$ YEARS

As for previous knowledge, these questions are ones where the answer to the question is not explicitly included in the text. The speller must use their own life experience and working memory to recall the answer. This may seem relatively straightforward. However, it can be complicated for students with apraxia. One part of the process involves memory storage, and the other is related to memory retrieval. Each process has several steps, such as encoding, consolidation, and retrieval. Furthermore, both short-term and long-term memory are involved as the student has to relate new information from the lesson to prior knowledge and experiences. This linking of ideas and information stored in the brain is a complex process and therefore is considered a much higher cognitive demand on the continuum. Possible examples of previous knowledge questions from this lesson would be:

> (Prior knowledge) What would be another word or way to describe "unparalleled"?

> (exceptional, unequaled, can't be matched, etc.)
> (Prior knowledge) Name another field of science.

The next step up the cognitive continuum involves open-ended questions, which are color-coded pink. They are questions that only the speller knows the answer to before they start to spell it out. This is the beginning of Speller's Method becoming a form of communication! Often emotions run high as spellers emerge into this level of the cognitive continuum, and the dysregulation which can come from the excitement does complicate it at times. But the pressure to perform is alleviated with practice and by starting with short one-word open responses. The speller will begin to develop the confidence and motor planning ability to spell longer and longer open answers. An example of what we call a "tight open" question would be the following:

> (Open) In a word, how do you think Stephen felt the day he was given the ALS diagnosis?

An example of a "broader open" question would be this:

> (Open) Stephen wanted his legacy to be that black holes aren't all black. This discovery has unalterably changed the world he's leaving behind. What might you want your legacy to be at the end of your life?

At this point in the speller's journey, we focus on the final step of the cognitive continuum—creative writing. This is where a student is spelling openly in complete sentences and is formulating paragraphs of novel content based on a writing prompt. We proceed through open questions scaffolded along the premise of Bloom's Taxonomy, each step requiring a bit more executive attention than the previous. An example of a creative writing question that we might ask at the end of the complete Stephen Hawking lesson would be:

> (Open) Compare and contrast your experience learning the Spellers Method to Stephen Hawking's lifelong learning of AAC. How do you think he felt with each new acquisition phase when his ALS progressed and he lost more muscle control? How did the acquisition phase of the Spellers Method feel to you? What insights have you developed from reflecting on both of your journeys?

EXECUTIVE ATTENTION

Executive attention is the ability to hold a thought (or answer) in your mind while organizing your body to do a motor task. The best example everyone can relate to is when you walk into the kitchen to get something but can't remember what you went there for. Holding on to our idea while executing a series of muscle movements can be difficult when our bodies and brains multitask. Those with autism and apraxia are also experiencing differences in sensory processing, which impact their motor output. As they progress along the motor and cognitive continuums during the acquisition phase of spelling, they also train their executive attention. They start by simply holding on to the letters of the word they are trying to spell. Then they must hold on to the answers to questions in single words or sentences while they spell them out, letter by letter, to communicate their ideas. The amount of neural firing increases within the brain as the cognitive demand increases: the more complex the cognitive demand, the more executive attention is required.

This is something we all learn to do when starting to learn a new motor skill. Take driving a car, for example. When you first got behind the wheel, you had to put all your concentration into the motor sequences needed to drive. You probably found it challenging to carry on a conversation with your passenger at the same time as looking in the rearview mirror to parallel park. If the weather was bad, you turned down the radio to reduce the cognitive demand because you needed to focus all your attention on the road. If you needed to quickly brake or swerve to avoid a skidding car, you didn't want to be distracted by the music. In those first few weeks of learning to drive a car, you were building your executive attention. Today, however, you can listen to a podcast, talk with multiple people in the car, or engage in a conference call on your phone (on speaker phone or hands-free, of course!), all while driving yourself to work. You navigate new traffic patterns daily but do not have to put conscious, deliberate thought into doing the muscle movements. You have mastered both the executive attention and the praxis involved in driving.

Your speller needs to work on this same skill set. They can't necessarily hold on to all of their thoughts while organizing their body to spell simultaneously. They have the ideas in their brain—and complex ones at that!—but once they start planning, sequencing, and organizing their motor to initiate spelling (the motor skill), they often struggle with executing it all. This is another reason why we prompt. We are there to give their bodies direction so they can succeed during this learning/acquisition phase. You might even think of practitioners as the GPS or Google Maps app for their apraxic bodies.

One of the ways we gradually increase the cognitive demand and associated executive attention is by writing questions based on Bloom's Taxonomy. This hierarchy has been used for generations in the academic setting, and we find it helpful in structuring lesson questions.

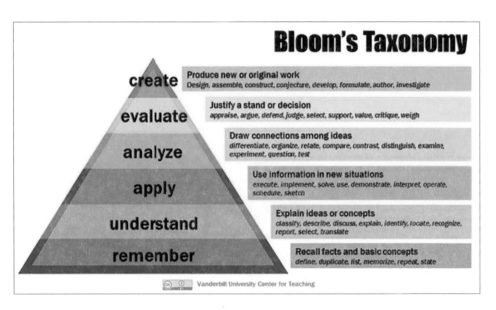

Bloom's Taxonomy

create — Produce new or original work
Design, assemble, construct, conjecture, develop, formulate, author, investigate

evaluate — Justify a stand or decision
appraise, argue, defend, judge, select, support, value, critique, weigh

analyze — Draw connections among ideas
differentiate, organize, relate, compare, contrast, distinguish, examine, experiment, question, test

apply — Use information in new situations
execute, implement, solve, use, demonstrate, interpret, operate, schedule, sketch

understand — Explain ideas or concepts
classify, describe, discuss, explain, identify, locate, recognize, report, select, translate

remember — Recall facts and basic concepts
define, duplicate, list, memorize, repeat, state

Vanderbilt University Center for Teaching

Each question in a lesson falls under one of these categories. Early in the journey, new spellers work on building their motor skills by recalling facts and basic concepts through known questions. This is the bottom tier of Bloom's Taxonomy. The CP needs to know the answer to provide the proper letterboard (when working on the three boards). They also need to know the answer so the CP can prompt the speller's eyes to get to the letter on the board to poke it. Spelling practice needs to continue this way to improve motor skills and accuracy.

When the practitioner or CP feels the speller's motor skills and accuracy have improved on the three letterboards, they will first increase the motor demand by going to the next letterboard on the motor continuum before increasing the cognitive demand. That's because the speller is still in the acquisition phase, and we need to build a solid foundation. Moving too quickly through the letterboards or question types will increase the risk of dysregulation and influencing. We aim to support the speller's regulation, so slow and steady wins the race here.

Once the speller is accurately spelling known answers on the 26 stencil, we will add semi-open questions, which are still part of the recall and remember tier on Bloom's taxonomy. Once they've mastered semi-opens, they can begin to answer open questions. This is when we start slowly moving up Bloom's Taxonomy. Here is a sample list of open questions in increasing complexity according to Bloom's paradigm:

Bloom's 1 - Recall: What was Stephen Hawking diagnosed with at the age of 21?

Bloom's 2 - Understand: Identify an emotion you think Stephen Hawking probably felt at the moment of his ALS diagnosis.

Bloom's 3 - Apply: Create an acrostic poem with the name "Hawking."

Bloom's 4 - Analyze: Compare your acquisition phase in Spellers Method to Stephen's ongoing acquisition phases each time he lost more muscle control and needed to change his access point for AAC.

Bloom's 5 - Evaluate: Defend how Stephen's example of how having a motor disability never meant he had a cognitive one is a similar experience to having motor apraxia and being a nonspeaker.

Bloom's 6 - Create: Stephen wanted his legacy to be that black holes aren't all black. This discovery has unalterably changed the world he's leaving behind. What might you want your legacy to be at the end of your life?

In summary, the takeaway message is that not all open questions are equivalent. Some require more executive attention than others, and consideration must be given to that fact, especially when spellers are emerging into open communication. Rushing students to that phase before building solid motor planning skills (scanning, finding, holding their visual fixation, and poking the letters cleanly and accurately) is imperative to support the more robust cognitive output we aim for with the Spellers Method as a communication technique. Working with a trained practitioner in a spelling methodology is highly recommended to ensure you keep moving steadily forward but avoid accidentally creating too big of a motor or cognitive challenge by skipping over critical steps.

ACQUISITION PHASE VERSUS APPLICATION PHASE

So what do we mean when we use terms like *acquisition phase* and *application phase*? The acquisition phase means anytime that we are learning or acquiring new skills. In spelling methods, the new skills being learned are the motor skills, including the ocular motor skills, needed to poke the letters accurately to spell. Prompting is used during the acquisition phase to help the speller learn these skills, and we fade the prompts as the speller builds the intentional motor skills. Because prompting is used, we can only ask the "known" and "math" questions in the lesson. Once the speller builds their motor skills, has moved to the 26-letter board, and prompting is reduced, we can shift to the semi-open questions. We continue to practice and build motor skills as frequently as possible. Practice is the key. Families often ask how they can progress fastest, and we always say, "Practice, practice, practice!"

The application phase occurs when spellers are fluent. They have already transitioned to a 26-letter board (stencil or foam) and have developed strong motor skills, so gestural and directional prompts are no longer needed. (The CP can still use initiation, eye, and continuation prompts during this phase.) Spellers in the application phase can demonstrate their knowledge and comprehension at this point in the spelling process. Their eyes are now moving to the letters they want, and their arm is following the eyes as they shift from letter to letter. The timing, coordination, and accuracy have improved significantly. The speller can answer open questions and begins to develop the endurance and stamina needed to answer creative writing questions and describe things in detail. This is an exciting process for everyone. The speller can demonstrate their knowledge consistently and reliably and, even more importantly, have conversations with family members or peers.

We have now hit the next stage of the spelling journey, and practice with lessons is just as crucial as during the first spelling session. Just because you won the competition doesn't mean you stop practicing. No! You continue to refine your skills to continue to improve and improve. The same is for spelling. Perhaps the speller has goals to go to college, type independently, have multiple communication partners, and advocate for other spellers by offering to speak at conferences. These goals require individualized attention and skills that need to be refined. Stay tuned. That's coming up next!

10

The Four Types of Movement

Science Alert: For those without any background in science, keep the glossary section of the handbook tabbed while you read through this section. Though we have tried to keep concepts simple, the terminology alone can be daunting to new families. Dana and DM have relied on their years of clinical experience to navigate the clinical research and the application of that research to the Spellers Method. Hopefully, this section feels digestible to even the non-scientifically-minded reader.

We engage in our typical daily routines, and most don't even think twice about how our brain and body make this happen. We take for granted our ability to move intentionally, and many times, we take for granted the ability of our speller's body to move intentionally as well.

Our bodies can move in four different ways. Movement originates from the brain's motor cortex, which is located in the frontal lobe. The first type of movement is purposeful or intentional movement, and it's what we referred to earlier as the process of praxis. This type of movement is initiated in the brain's frontal lobe because it requires conscious thought. We have to think through these movements as we coordinate our bodies and adjust when things don't go as planned. As we continue to practice movement, neural pathways are being built so that we don't have to put so much thought and focus into the movement for the rest of our lives once these connections are made and are myelinated.

> **Dana:** Myelin is an insulating layer, or sheath, that forms around nerves, including those in the brain and spinal cord. It is made up of protein and fatty substances. When neural pathways are *myelinated,* all the synaptic connections are covered in a myelin sheath, allowing the electrical impulses to transmit quickly and efficiently along the nerve cells. In the case of forming new neural pathways for movement, this also results in more efficient motor output. The more you practice a particular motor action, the more you fire impulses along the same neural pathway. The more times that pathway fires together, the more it wires together. As it wires together, it develops the myelin sheath and becomes even more efficient!

We no longer have to think about each step as they have become automatic. Automatic movements, the second type of movement, occur without conscious thought. We rely on our bodies moving automatically so we can do what we need throughout the day without thinking about it. Have you ever driven to work and not remembered how you got there because you had been thinking about a potentially stressful situation? Your safety was 100 percent due to your automatic movements in that situation. When you practice a movement (e.g., driving to work) repeatedly, it will become automatic. Automatic movement is a "good" thing for the most part. It makes us as efficient as possible. However, automatic movements for those with apraxia can get complicated, and we're about to find out why.

The last two types of movement include reflexive movement and impulsive movement. Both these movements are involuntary, and we do not consciously think about making these movements. Reflexive movement helps us to build our gross motor skills when we are infants as we progress through the developmental stages. Reflexive movements also protect us from dangerous situations, hopefully preventing us from getting hurt. We are born with various types of "primitive reflexes." These reflexes include oral reflexes, which help initiate the sucking movement to nourish us. The Moro reflex occurs when the infant's body is out of balance, and the grasping reflex occurs when there is pressure put on the palm of the infant's hand. All of these examples disappear as the infant develops and are replaced by voluntary movement. It is important to note that reflexive movement patterns can be retained, meaning that they don't disappear. Retained reflexes can then disrupt voluntary or intentional movement, and many individuals with autism have retained reflexes. Specific details on reflex integration are beyond the scope of this book. However, it is important to consider and talk with your occupational therapist if you have questions.

Reflexive movements that keep us safe continue through life. For example, if we are cooking and accidentally get too close to the pot of boiling water, we will immediately take our hands away. We don't stop to think about this action. If we did, we would for sure be burned! This sensory information (hot temperature felt on the skin) doesn't make it up to the "thinking" part of our brain. It only makes it to our spinal cord and triggers our hand movement quickly because the body is in danger. Impulsive movement is also involuntary but is triggered differently.

When we experience sensory overload or intense emotion, our bodies respond impulsively. If we think about our spellers, we know that individuals with autism may have sensory differences and can be over-or under-responsive to sensory stimuli. The anticipation of a sensory experience can also trigger anxiety. Because of the sensory overload (e.g., loud environment) plus the emotion (e.g., fear), the speller is more likely to be impulsive with their body. The impulsive response is often self-injury or injury toward others. When it happens, emotions run high for everyone in the room. The key here is to remember that impulsive movement is *involuntary*. It isn't an intentional reaction when the speller grabs your hair or pinches, bites, or kicks. Often, we jump to conclusions that may or may not be accurate.

Many spellers will demonstrate impulsive behavior and then spell that it was not what they wanted to do. Impulsive movement can be challenging. However, it also highlights our essential role as coregulators. If the speller is dysregulated in any way, our first goal should always be regulation. This will help with the impulsivity the speller desperately tries to avoid.

Unfortunately, so many spellers aren't supported to regulate, which results in these impulsive movements happening over and over. We know that when a movement occurs repeatedly, that movement becomes myelinated or automatic. Whenever a flood of emotions or an overload in sensory input happens, impulsive movement will likely take over. We can't emphasize it enough: remember this isn't voluntary. When your speller reaches up to grab your hair or pinch your arm, these movements aren't because they don't want to spell with you or are trying to "escape" the task. It means that they need support to regulate their emotions and sensory input. The statement "all behavior is communication" used to be an accepted phrase. Now that we know so much more about the sensory-motor differences in those with autism, we actually understand that "behavior isn't *always* communication."

11

Sensory Processing and the Sensory-Motor Feedback Loop

Most of us know that autistic people have differences in processing sensory information from their environment. Sensory processing disorder (SPD) is only recognized in the DSM-V as a clinical manifestation of autism, not a stand-alone diagnosis. Parents and researchers continue to fight for those who don't have an autism diagnosis but struggle with processing sensory input. It wasn't until 2015 that SPD was added under autism and more professionals took it seriously. When it comes to nonspeaking autism, sensory-motor differences impact an individual's ability to move their body efficiently. Simply put, sensory information from our environment comes into our brain through the sensory receptors and produces movements based on how our brain processes incoming sensory information. If there is a disruption in sensory processing, which there is for those with autism, it will inevitably disrupt the motor response.

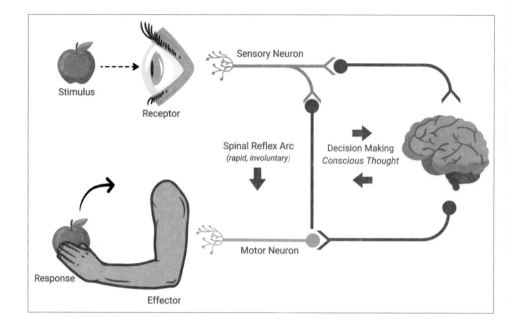

Here is a list of the sensory systems that we typically talk about:

- Proprioceptive system—Our body's ability to know where it is in space. We have proprioceptors in our muscles and joints that send information to the brain so we know how much force to use when we are holding something or how to position our body when rock climbing. When your proprioceptive system is not working effectively, you may seek out input and pressure to activate the proprioceptors.
- Vestibular system—Our sense of balance comes from the vestibular system. In conjunction with receptors in the inner ear and the visual system the goal of the vestibular system is to keep the body upright.
- Tactile system
- Auditory system
- Visual system
- Olfactory (smell) system
- Gustatory (taste) system

It's important to note that these systems all work together. We need our visual system to work with our proprioceptive system for efficiency with movement in space. Another sensory system known as interoception is a lesser-known sense but involves knowing how you feel inside your body. This includes emotional feelings and physical sensations such as hunger, thirst, the need to use the bathroom, etc.

For our spellers, the environment and its onslaught of sensory input significantly impact their regulation and ability to spell. Learning about your speller's sensory profile will help you better understand how to support your child. This will be useful not just with spelling but also in their everyday life.

We often assume that everyone processes sensory information the same way we do. But in reality, everyone processes sensory information differently, especially for those on the autism spectrum. In the case of neurotypical people, our nervous system is wired to adjust and self-regulate despite constant changes in incoming data as needed. We have the connection between our brain and our body to make those pivots and take action to self-regulate. Those with apraxia and autism have a disruption in that connection (Torres & Whyatt, 2020) due to inefficient sensory processing and the neuro-motor connection. They have more difficulty making those adjustments and filtering through the stimuli around them.

If a person's neuroreceptors are overloaded and the incoming sensory information is overwhelming, the motor response will often be impulsive with possible self-injurious or injurious toward others. If the messages sent from the neuroreceptors to the brain are even slightly disrupted, the motor output will be inefficient. Elizabeth Torres refers to this disruption as excess "noise" in the system (Torres et al, 2013). She talks about how the incoming sensory information coming into the brain becomes random, and the brain can't filter out unnecessary input. The result is a broken sensory-motor feedback loop which significantly impacts how we control our bodies and learn new motor movements.

The *CliffsNote* version of the above section is that a person with difficulties in sensory processing will, by definition, have difficulties in their motor output. You can learn more about sensory-motor feedback by reading Elizabeth Torres's work.

SENSORY PROFILES

Many parents come to us and tell us that their child has strengths in certain sensory processing areas. For example, they often say, "My child is a visual learner." Parents make this conclusion based on what they observe their child doing. The child may love scrolling through pictures or YouTube, or spend long periods of time visually examining something in front of them. This same child might have visual schedules all over the house because their parents have noticed that seeing the steps of a task rather than just hearing them has been a more effective teaching strategy.

The truth is, all of us are multisensory learners and so is your child! We know that our nonspeakers learn in many different ways, not just the one sensory system they seem to prefer. We have found that many spellers are auditory and kinesthetic learners as well. It might seem confusing to parents at first because they don't "look" like they are listening when they are moving all around the therapy room, however many of our spellers are taking in information even when we don't think they are.

> **Dana:** One of my clients who was in an AP high school algebra class with his CP would routinely try to leave the classroom just before class would start. His CP was doing all he could to coach the student back into the classroom because the student had spelled how much he loved algebra. Finally, the CP asked why he kept trying to leave and the speller spelled "I HEAR BETTER AT THE END OF THE HALLWAY." What??! Yes! This student heard the teacher best when he was outside the classroom and

down at the other end of the hallway. It was too over-whelming for his auditory system to be sitting directly in the classroom.

Apraxia does make the body do things the person doesn't want to do and, in the example above, the CP thought the student's body was doing something impulsive by leaving the classroom. Yet, it was about the sensory profile of the student and how he learns best. This is one of the reasons why in our sessions we continue to read the lesson even if the student doesn't "look" like they are listening. We continue to read even if they are down the hall, outside of the room, or singing scripted lyrics to us as we speak. We will say to parents, "Neurotypicals are often terrible listeners because we talk too much. We are often just waiting for our turn to speak, so we aren't truly paying attention to what's being said. Our nonspeakers, on the other hand, take in *everything* all the time. This is how they have learned a lot of what they know."

When we talk with parents about their child's sensory-motor profile, we are referring to the things that their bodies do to move toward a more regulated state. It may seem strange to think that if your son or daughter cannot stop moving their body, they might be doing this to help themselves regulate. In fact, it looks like they are significantly dysregulated. What is happening is that their body has a higher threshold for a certain amount of specific sensory input, so they may need *more* of one thing to reach their threshold.

In other sensory-motor profiles, we observe the child avoiding certain types of sensory input, and that is because they have a lower threshold for that specific input. To make things even more compli-cated, a child can be a sensory seeker in one area but avoid other types of sensory input in other areas. If you think about it, we also have a sensory-motor profile, and you may need a higher threshold of certain sensory input but avoid other types of input. Sensory-motor profiles also change as we age. We can all think about times in our life when we would seek out sensory stimuli, and now we wouldn't engage in the same activity, and we might even avoid it. For example, as a young person, roller coasters and theme parks may have been your jam, but now even thinking about getting on a roller coaster makes you nauseous. Sitting in the front row at a concert once excited you, but now being close to so many people and the amount of auditory stimulation for hours makes you cringe.

The difference between our sensory-motor system and your child's sensory-motor system is that their brain processes the incoming sensory information much differently and often inefficiently. As a result, the motor output is what we observe: impulsivity, inability to sit, covering their ears, constant climbing, can't stop their body, or having difficulty starting a task. Figuring out the ever-changing sensory-motor profile of your child can be challenging, let alone trying to figure out how to support them best.

Below we have described several profiles and provided suggestions on supporting their regulation. However, working with a Spellers Method practitioner or an occupational therapist can give you some much-needed insight into their individual sensory-motor profile, especially as things change. It is important to note that the following profiles and suggestions are meant to be just that: suggestions only. Getting a complete understanding and recommendations specific to your speller from an occupational therapist or Spellers Method practitioner is important.

KINESTHETIC-SEEKING BODIES

Kinesthetically seeking spellers tend to want to touch or handle everything in sight. Some may pick up an item and play with it; some may pick it up and put it in their mouths; others may lick it. Some also have difficulty keeping their bodies in the chair. Some put everything in their mouths because they need oral stimulation and deep pressure in their jaw or to explore the space. Spellers who touch everything in the room need input to help better "understand" the area. It's giving them information that other sensory systems may not be giving them.

Suggestions for spellers that are kinesthetic seekers include:

- Crunchy, cold, chewy foods to keep their mouths busy and to give input.
- Body engagers—An activity that requires intentional motor (usually involving the hands) to help engage the student's mind and hands and will help them remain seated in the chair. Examples of body engagers include:
  - Rubix cube
  - Sticker by Number book
  - Drawing
  - Pop It
  - Bubble rap

PROPRIOCEPTIVE-SEEKING BODIES

Spellers seeking proprioception tend to be "intense," meaning they squeeze hard on anything they touch. They will also squeeze their bodies into small areas and love jumping, crashing, or "roughhouse." These spellers may need additional deep pressure before or during a spelling session to support regulation.

Other suggestions include the following:

- Deep pressure on arms and shoulders to help ground the speller
- Lifting a medicine ball and tossing it ten times
- Weighted blanket or lap pad
- Using rhythm along with deep pressure

IMPULSIVE BODIES

Spellers whose bodies are impulsive have a difficult time with inhibition. With apraxia, we know that initiation is very challenging, but inhibiting the body can be just as difficult for some. Sometimes spellers will reach up and grab the practitioner's hair, kick, pinch, or throw whatever object is in front of them. These are all impulsive movements and are not intentional. Remember from the previous section that impulsive movement is triggered by emotions, sensory experiences, or both. When spelling, spellers can feel a lot of emotion, and if there is sensory input that is too much for them, this will often cause some impulsive bodies to jump up, possibly try and leave the room, or reach over and grab your shirt. The most important thing to remember, which is also the most challenging in the moment, is that the speller wants to do something other than what they are doing.

The difficult thing about impulsive bodies is that they know they might have hurt the practitioner or parent or shouldn't be running into traffic, but they can't stop themselves. They then feel anxious, stressed, or sad, and what does that do? Cause more impulsive movement because of the flood of emotions! The best thing we can do to support spellers in this situation is to reduce stress, anxiety, and overall emotions. Right, we know, easier said than done! In later chapters, we have covered regulation and coregulation, so fear not; we will not leave you without strategies.

SENSORY-AVOIDING BODIES

Some sensory input can be so strong to spellers that it actually causes pain. For those of us without sensory processing challenges, we don't often stop to think that others around us might perceive sensory input differently than we do. We take it for granted that everyone senses the same. We must take spellers who avoid sensory input seriously and not say things like it's "just a little noise" when covering their ears. Some spellers have described the brush of another person's hand on their arm as burning, tingling, and intense pain. Others have talked about sounds like a freight train was crossing in front of them. Surely you can imagine the emotions and anxiety that come from that.

If you notice that spellers are tactile defensive (avoiding light touch), auditorily defensive, or visually defensive, it's vital to note. Hand over hand will cause dysregulation, as will loud voices or spaces. Many people moving around in a room will also be difficult for the speller to keep regulated.

Suggestions to support sensory defensive spellers:

- Speaking softly (whispering) and using a lower tone helps.
- Avoid hand over hand or touching their body.
- Dimming the lights or spelling in a room with natural light.

12

Building Intentional Movement

We all learn new motor movements through a process called neuro-plasticity. Neuroplasticity, as defined by the Oxford dictionary, is the ability of the brain to form and reorganize synaptic connections in response to learning, experience, or after an injury. One of the reasons why we are all encouraged to take up a new sport or hobby, build something, or do a puzzle is because this helps us build new connections in our brain and keeps it healthy.

Those with apraxia can also build new pathways and connections through this same process of neuroplasticity. How does this happen? The exact same way as anyone else—practicing the movement pattern over and over. This can be challenging when the body isn't cooperating. The sensory-motor profiles of our clients are all so different. If a speller has a sensory-motor profile that is more impulsive, they may need more coaching and practice. Those with less impulsivity may acquire the intentional movement skills quicker. There isn't any "ideal" profile to progress quicker. We were all given a certain body and sensory-motor profile and some of us have to work harder than others to get things together.

So how do we "coach the motor"? Well, the first thing that absolutely has to happen is we presume competence. Remember that part of presuming competence is that we 100 percent believe that the individual we are talking to understands what we are asking of them even if they don't look like they are listening or look like they understand. This can be a hurdle for some because we have to forget the years of being told that they don't understand. We also believe that listening should "look" a certain way (i.e., the child stills their body, isn't fidgeting with anything, and perhaps makes eye contact) but they don't look like they are listening! It's a mindset shift we all have to make in order to become successful motor coaches.

The second thing we need to do is presume competence in their body. This means that we believe they want to control their body better. They want to be able to do things that are asked of them. When we can presume competence all around, we can then regulate ourselves better when they bolt toward the door, or when their mouth says "No!" or when they don't move from the chair. This is when we need to start to coach the motor.

13

Coaching the Motor

Typically, when we use the term "task analysis" our mind may go to behavioral interventions. Yes, that is a term ABA therapists use; however, a task analysis in this case is related to breaking down a motor skill into many small steps. We do this so that we can give the speller's body direction in order to complete the task rather than giving them one instruction (e.g., "Wash your hands") or essentially telling them the end goal. Think of motor coaching as the same as prompting when you're practicing spelling. You are using prompts to help their body get to the letter.

We want the speller to go sit in the chair to practice spelling. Many people would simply say "Go sit in the chair so we can spell." This isn't wrong; however, the speller may need more support to get their body started. Remember, initiation is the most challenging part of getting the body to complete a task. When we coach the motor, the verbiage can go something like this:

1. Get your eyes on the chair—when we can get their eyes to the target, this helps with initiation because our eyes direct our body.
2. Turn your body to the chair (if they are turned around).
3. Bring your foot forward, bring your other foot forward (continue with this until they gain the momentum to walk toward the chair).
4. As they get to the chair you can say "turn your body" so they are facing away from the chair.
5. Bend your knees.
6. Push your hips back.
7. Sit.

This may seem extreme and for some spellers it's not necessary to break it down so much. Some don't need this much coaching and their challenge is more related to initiating their body to start the movement. Others will need step by step coaching to get their body to complete the task. For the caregiver it takes time to make this verbiage a natural part of your vocabulary, but it will become very natural the more that you practice. You will quickly see how much this helps your speller, which will give you more confidence and assurance that this is what they need from you.

14

Motor Differences and Motor Loops

A *motor loop* is a term we use to describe a repetitive movement that may or may not be intentional. It is an automatic movement that has been practiced over and over which has resulted in a well-myelinated neural pathway between the brain and the moving body part(s).

A motor loop can be a gross motor movement (e.g., grabbing mom's cell phone and handing it back to her every time she sets it down) or a fine motor movement (e.g., repeating a phrase over and over again, saying "All done" or "Time to go home"). Often a loop starts because of a feeling or an emotion. For example, when an unreliable speaker repeatedly states that they are going to lunch after their spelling session—"First spelling, then lunch"—over and over, this is a loop. They may lean into your face, as if they're asking you to acknowledge what they have said. When you do acknowledge with either a head nod or a verbal response, they will go back to spelling a few words. Moments later, however, they jump back into their loop again. They lean in, repeat their phrase, wait for your acknowledgement, and then go back to spelling. This is an example of a motor loop. The speller often needs another person to close their loop in the form of the CP acknowledging it, saying a particular phrase, or confirming yes or no to the speller. If they try to ignore the speller's loop oftentimes the speller's arousal level starts to go up and it may lead to dysregulation.

Another example would be when the parent or caregiver is talking with another person the child picks up mom's purse and gives it to her. Mom says, "It's not time to go yet, we just started." A few seconds later the speller picks up the purse again and gives it to his mom. Again, mom says, "It's not time yet." It seems as though the child is trying to communicate that they want to leave; however, as we have learned with apraxia, body movements may not be what they seem. If every time a speller does A (hands mom the purse) and we respond with B (saying "It's not time yet"), we start to make these loops more permanent. Think of it like creating tire paths in a muddy dirt road. The more we drive in the same tire treads the more permanent those pathways become.

So how do motor loops start in the first place? Well, as we learned earlier, the more we practice a movement, the more automatic it becomes. As we continue to develop and we practice gross and fine motor skills, our bodies become very efficient at moving around. An example of a motor loop that a non-apraxic person might use would be this: you may walk by a stranger on the street and, without even thinking, you make eye contact so you say, "Hey, how are you?" the other person responds by saying "Good, thanks!" and you both continue walking in your opposite directions. These are motor loops that we have practiced as we built our social repertoire. It's not until that loop is scrambled that we have to put actual thought into it. For example, after you asked how the person is doing, if instead of responding with a simple "Fine, thanks!" they stopped walking and went into a long dialogue about how their day has started out terribly, their car needs a new battery, their lunch dropped on the sidewalk, etc., your brain would send you an alert. What is happening here?

Pay attention. This stranger just went off the motor loop script. Here you were just unconsciously showing good social etiquette when this guy scrambled your motor plan. Now you're going to be late for work because you are involved in a conversation that you weren't expecting! That might teach your brain to not unconsciously ask someone "How are you?" tomorrow.

For apraxic bodies, motor loops can be extremely frustrating but they can also be a strategy for regulation. Many spellers have talked about loops that are frustrating and loops that help to calm. Here are just a couple of quotes from self-advocates on the topic of loops:

> Calling a loop a "loop" can demean its recharging power because then it can be viewed as negative. I like it when [someone] asks me whether I want help breaking an impulsive action. That way I am in control of my purposefulness.—Jordyn Pallett

> If I had not been taught how to control my hand enough to type with my index finger on a keyboard, iPad or letterboard, my ideas, jokes and thoughts would have been known only to myself. This is how it is for thousands of people with autism who cannot communicate. —Ido Kedar

> My body does not listen to my brain. It has many minds of its own. My wish is for the world to understand this. Knowing this makes loads of difference for people who are autistic like me.—Elliot Sylvester

Traditional therapies for autism focus on repetition (a.k.a. practicing) of motor movements over and over again. Speech therapists work on articulation, forming words, and using augmentative and alternative communication (AAC) devices. In an effort to support the child with communication they have them practice the same patterns (words or pointing to icons) over and over again. If done without actually coaching the child's body or motor, the result can be that the child has developed some automatic movements. They will often touch the icons unintentionally.

Remember that those with apraxia have significant difficulty initiating and inhibiting movement. So, if they want to use their device and they've practiced a certain pattern many times (e.g., "I want more juice") their body will go to each of those icons even when they don't want juice. Other therapies focus on motor skills such as following a point, pushing a car back and forth, or other play patterns that are considered "socially appropriate." These may seem purposeful at first (even though they are arguably ableist as well) but once learned, it can be difficult to inhibit these movement patterns because of apraxia. One of the main reasons we don't practice spelling the same words repeatedly or do the same lesson more than once in Spellers Method is because we want to constantly work on purposeful movement and not create loops. When you learned to drive a car, you learned to operate the machine, not memorize the traffic patterns that day and navigate those exact same traffic patterns every single day. Pointing to letters becomes automated, but the sequence of the letters and the words they spell out must remain consistently novel.

So how do we break the automatic patterns or motor loops that are causing the body to get "stuck"? We focus on building intentional movement patterns rather than focusing on the loop itself. Those with apraxia need support to engage their bodies in any intentional activity. In fact, most report that they'd prefer to be doing something intentional with their bodies. When their body is not engaged that is when we see more loops happen.

When we are in a spelling session it's easier to get the spellers body to move intentionally because spelling is intentional movement. When a family is in the car on the way to grandma's house your child may be stuck in a verbal loop or stuck in a loop that includes throwing a toy over and over again. Coaching your child to do something purposeful with their body is the best way to break the loop. It's important to remember these loops didn't develop in a day or two so breaking them isn't going to happen in a day. It's about consistency and recognizing that your child is in a loop and you may be a part of it. Scrambling or breaking the loop will happen but it takes time.

> **Dana**: The topic of motor loops often comes up during the first session with a new speller because motor loops can be triggered by emotions. The session is typically full of emotions from everyone in the room! My goal is to get the speller engaged in the intentional movement of spelling because that is a very effective way to move past the loop and begin to break or scramble the loop. It's also a great opportunity to talk with parents about loops that are purposeful and loops that may not be and result in the speller getting stuck.

Not only should parents and professionals become curious about the motor differences displayed in nonspeakers, but we must also advocate for a nonspeaker's right to choose which motor differences should be respected and which motor differences they would like support in overcoming, whether temporarily or more permanently. For example, in terms of using a letterboard or keyboard to communicate, there are often motor differences that pose challenges for students who are trying to develop fluency. Assuming that most new spellers do want access to effective communication, the question then is: Should motor loops be interrupted in non-fluent spellers in order to help them develop more purposeful motor actions such as pointing and spelling? We think yes, but it must be done with a tremendous amount of respect, dignity, and communication with the speller.

Through the lens of neurodiversity rights advocates, behaviors of the people who would ordinarily be classified as non-neurotypical are simply normal expressions of human function rather than disorders to be diagnosed and treated. Though this perspective has merit, is honoring, and is definitely person-centered, it doesn't address the fact that many nonspeakers do want help sometimes overcoming impulsive, repetitive motor actions. Helping a speller in a way that honors their individual differences but also supports their acquisition of effective communication is of critical importance as well as a basic right. Once the nonspeaker can spell fluently, they naturally become the subject matter expert who drives their parent or practitioner's support.

In the meantime, we adhere to the least dangerous assumption in case we are wrong about the speller's desire whether to break a loop or not. We also have the wisdom of already fluent typers and spellers who guide us. Their advice is that not myelinating any more loops that interrupt other, more needed intentional motor plans, ultimately leads to greater autonomy for the speller down the road. More motor control means more ability to inhibit impulses. More impulse inhibition leads to more community access. More community access leads to more friendships, more opportunities, and more autonomy.

In the meantime, while we await and/or pioneer further research into the neurobiological etiology of autism, apraxia, and the sensory-motor differences expressed within these conditions let us remember this quote from Albert Einstein: "Not everything that counts can be counted and not everything that is counted counts." Sometimes we have to start back at the beginning, and in this case by reconsidering the criteria used to diagnose autism in the first place, and propose a course adjustment.

15
Regulation

The word *regulation* comes up a lot in the field of autism, and in the world of spelling you'll often see it added to the title of the communication partner, making them a CRP, or communication *regulation* partner. The pricelessness of an effective communication partner is deeply rooted in their ability to regulate the speller, even more than in their ability to switch boards or prompt smoothly. So what is this concept of regulation and how does someone improve their ability to regulate themselves and others?

In the simplest terms, regulation means managing yourself. It's having the ability to recognize your internal needs, make good decisions in the moment, and respond to your emotions in adaptive ways. When regulated, a person feels a sense of balance. This state can be described as feeling calm, alert, ready and available for engaging with others.

Imagine walking into a room of spellers. With a quick scan of the eye, the first thing you might notice is each speller's arousal level.

Arousal levels are the degree of alertness or responsiveness to stimuli. In a room full of spellers there is usually a lot of stimuli . . . moving bodies, vocalizations or scripting, various body positions on furniture, etc. You can quickly see which students are hyperresponsive to the stimuli in the room and which are hypo-responsive.

Arousal levels are controlled in your brain by what's called the reticular activating system (RAS). The ability of the RAS to filter stimuli so your nervous system doesn't get overwhelmed is influenced by emotions, sensory input, and neurotransmitters. This area is also involved in the body's "fight, flight, or freeze" response. It's important to remember that those with sensory processing differences tend to respond differently to the sensory input around them. They will not filter the environmental stimuli the same way as we do. Moreover, emotions—even positive ones—can tip their arousal level into hyperdrive very easily.

The ability to regulate oneself depends on many things, but most notably on that ability to process incoming sensory information. Autistics have a lot of difficulty in this area. That said, none of us were born with the ability to self-regulate. Our parents and caregivers coregulated with us until we could do so ourselves. So, the interdependence human beings share to maintain their own internal states of regulation is somewhat innate.

We know we're preaching to the choir when we say your speller's neurological system may be sensitive to various things in the environment. No kidding, right? Undoubtedly, you've spent years trying to avoid all the triggers that might dysregulate them so you could navigate social situations and life in general. It's what we do as parents, especially when trying to prevent a meltdown. So, let's talk a little bit about what's happening inside the body when their nervous system (or yours) gets triggered.

POLYVAGAL THEORY

World-renowned researcher Dr. Stephen Porges coined the term *neuroception* back in 1994. He describes it as the process by which our reptilian or primitive brain receives incoming sensory information from our environment. This information tells us whether the situation at hand is safe or not. Based on this information, our body responds in several different ways. However, the trouble with neuroception is that it can give faulty information to our brains.

Dr. Porges's work, known as the Polyvagal Theory, focuses on the vagus nerve, one of the twelve cranial nerves. The word *vagus* means "wandering" in Latin. It is appropriately named because it is the longest cranial nerve in the body. It runs from the brain stem (the primitive brain) to the large intestine. It's responsible for all sorts of automatic activities like heart rate, breathing, digestion, and reflexive actions such as sneezing, swallowing, and vomiting. It seems pretty important, right? We agree.

What's interesting about cranial nerves is that some have sensory functions, meaning they take in sensory information and send it to the brain. Others have motor functions, meaning they are responsible for moving specific muscles or making glands work appropriately. The vagus nerve is a special one. It is the one cranial nerve that has *both* sensory and motor functions. As such, one of its most important functions is its pivotal role in activating part of the autonomic nervous system.

Through the process of neuroception and the action of the vagus nerve, our brain is sent signals about the environment. This activates the autonomic nervous system and results in our body entering one of three physiological states. When this happens, a person's level of arousal goes up or down accordingly, and their resulting social behavior changes dramatically. This is true for all human beings, by the way, not just our spellers.

In 2018 Deb Dana visually described these three physiological states in what she called the "Autonomic Ladder" pictured here:

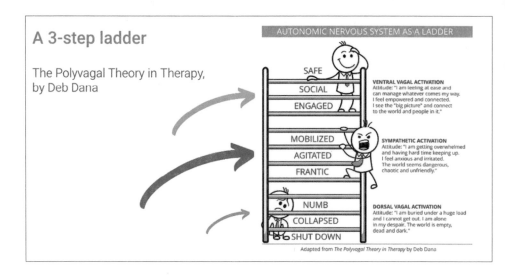

A 3-step ladder

The Polyvagal Theory in Therapy,
by Deb Dana

AUTONOMIC NERVOUS SYSTEM AS A LADDER

SAFE
SOCIAL
ENGAGED

VENTRAL VAGAL ACTIVATION
Attitude: "I am feeling at ease and can manage whatever comes my way. I feel empowered and connected. I see the "big picture" and connect to the world and people in it."

MOBILIZED
AGITATED
FRANTIC

SYMPATHETIC ACTIVATION
Attitude: "I am getting overwhelmed and having hard time keeping up. I feel anxious and irritated. The world seems dangerous, chaotic and unfriendly."

NUMB
COLLAPSED
SHUT DOWN

DORSAL VAGAL ACTIVATION
Attitude: "I am buried under a huge load and I cannot get out. I am alone in my despair. The world is empty, dead and dark."

Adapted from *The Polyvagal Theory in Therapy* by Deb Dana

When our nervous system receives information that puts us at the top of the ladder, we are put into a parasympathetic or ventral vagus state. This is where we feel most "like ourselves" and where all regulation, social engagement, and connection happens. We want both the speller and communication partner to be in this state while practicing their spelling lessons. The speller can tune into the activity, tune out most distractions, and is ready to learn.

When our nervous system receives information that it's being threatened or in danger, it moves us down the ladder, and the sympathetic nervous system becomes activated. The brain sends a signal that sends us into fight or flight mode. When this happens to a speller, they have two options: battle their way out of the situation or escape it entirely. Their heart rate speeds up, their breathing becomes shallower. If we are astute enough to notice the earliest signs of this happening to a speller, that's the best point to intervene by modeling strategies that reassure them (and their nervous system) back into the ventral vagus state. More on ways to do that in just a bit.

Alas, if strategies aren't employed, or those strategies prove to be ineffective, we may slide down the ladder to the point where the dorsal vagal state is activated. At this stage, our bodies become immobilized in fear. Spellers in this state might curl into a tight circle or roll into a ball on the floor and stop responding to anyone around them. Think of this as a "conservation" mode of sorts. It's pretty far down the evolutionary ladder, and it's meant to be protective. It's the nervous system's last-ditch effort to be safe. Note: it is *not* task avoidance or laziness.

In the autistic body, there are well-identified sensory perceptual differences. Accordingly, these differences often lead to faulty neuroception, or rather, misinterpretation of the environmental stimuli as threatening when it isn't. Sensory processing is dependent on the brain's ability to receive and interpret input from all of our senses: touch (tactile), taste (gustatory), hearing (auditory), sight (visual), smell (olfactory), spatial awareness (proprioception), balance (vestibular), and interoception (internal sensation awareness).

According to Leekam et al. 2007, 90 percent of children and adults with autism experience some disruption in sensory processing. Meanwhile, based on the exceptional research of Elizabeth Torres, we know that irregular neural connectivity is also associated with autism. This includes a reduction in the connections that facilitate sensory processing. In so many words, the sensory processing differences in autism frequently result in faulty neuroception.

So, what does this mean during your spelling sessions (and beyond)?

1. The nervous system of a nonspeaker receives signals that they are in danger even when they understand logically that there is no threat. Logic does not fix the faulty neuroception.
2. Their bodies can be more easily triggered into dysregulation because of this faulty neuroception.
3. How we meet our children in the moment of their dysregulation greatly impacts our ability to coregulate with them. In other words, put the proverbial oxygen mask on yourself first if they are dysregulated. This will help you coregulate with them.

4. In your spelling sessions don't forget this principle of altered neuroception even when your mind is telling you an old story. You might think your child is "misbehaving" or "doesn't want to spell" when really they are doing the very best they can to process the incoming sensory information and not completely shut down.

Just like a root system anchors a plant, we provide anchoring for the speller while serving as their CP. Through our own regulation and our ability to coregulate with them, we help create the neuroception of safety.

CREATING THE NEUROCEPTION OF SAFETY

In utero, the fetus's survival is carefully regulated by the mother through the umbilical cord. It delivers oxygen and nutrients, keeps the fetus feeling safe, warm, secure, and alive. After birth the helpless baby still needs all these things, so how does it get it?

There is actually a direct brain-to-brain link that connects the infant brain to the parent's brain. The parent's brain has the ability to regulate arousal in the infant. How it works is the mom or dad reads the baby's cues and adjusts their behavior to either up-regulate or down-regulate accordingly. What they're trying to achieve is that parasympathetic state where the baby's nervous system is "just right."

In the first year of life this starts out as a right-brain to right-brain connection. The right side of our brain is associated with intuitive thoughts and subjective thinking, usually triggered by nonverbal body language of someone else. Their tone of voice, their body language, their facial expressions, etc. gives us all the information we need. By the end of year one, the connection occurs from left-brain to left-brain too, which means the language centers are developed and become part of the coregulation process. At this point, the foundation is fully set for parental coregulation. There is deep neurological, psychological, and emotional circuitry that exists between parents and their children and this connection continues to grow as your child grows.

Some of you may be thinking that's good news, and others may be thinking it's bad.

The good news is that you, as the parent of a nonspeaker, are uniquely qualified to coregulate your autistic child. It's true. Genetically and neurologically, you're well suited for the job. Now don't worry if you feel like you feel inept at it sometimes. Or perhaps your spouse usually takes that role with your child. There are plenty of tools you can add to your coregulation toolbox to support productive spelling sessions. The point is, you are genetically wired for this gig. Congratulations! Now for the "how to."

COREGULATION

The process of coregulation involves being totally present together in the same moment. One partner helps to regulate another by responding contingently to that person's cues. Picture a newborn crying. You pick them up because you notice them flailing around in the crib. You immediately lower your voice into a soothing tone and start saying "Shhhhhh-hhhh-hhhh" as you bounce them gently up and down, then pull them in toward your chest and heartbeat. When they start to quiet a little, you might stop making sounds and sway gently back and forth in a rhythmic motion, carefully noticing which direction their arousal level is going. If they pick up the crying again you might resume the stronger bounces and vocal soothing. If they hush and nod off, you might give them a pacifier and return them to their crib. This is coregulation we've all either watched or participated in at some point.

Think also about the toddler who is enthusiastically running toward you but trips and falls face first onto the pavement. Startled, they look up at you first without making a sound. If you respond with

"Oh no!!! Are you okay?" they take their cue from you and start crying. If you respond with a big smile (even though you're praying they aren't really hurt) and say "Oops! You're okay!" they may grimace for a moment but they don't cry. Within seconds they're back running and laughing again. Coregulation for the "W" on that maneuver, mom and dad.

By using your grounded, calm presence and energy you help your partner feel competent, safe, and challenged in just the right amount. It is a dance! And the same is true for spelling sessions. As the CP, you create the energy in the room that hopefully grounds them and you. You use your voice and your prompting to set a tempo and rhythm that is just as effective as bouncing a newborn infant until they find themselves soothed in the safety of your motion. The speller's nervous system needs similar grounding so that their brain can focus on the motor planning required to spell, not be sending signals to escape the situation at hand.

When thinking about coregulation during spelling, the first tool is to make sure each partner is fulfilling a competent role. That means you should prep ahead of time. Know what your cognitive and motor goals are for the session, don't fly by the seat of your pants. Be sure to prompt your speller so they can achieve the goals you've set. Also be sure to assess your own self-regulation before you begin to practice together. You can't regulate someone else if you're not feeling regulated yourself. You know what they say on an airplane—you must put the oxygen mask on yourself before helping others. Same is true here for practicing spelling.

We often recommend you assess your own regulation state by giving yourself a number from 0–10. Let's assume 0 means you're so low on the arousal continuum you're practically sleep-walking and 10 would be so high on the arousal continuum you're having a panic attack or in full blown fight or flight. Think about what number would feel "just right" to you. A number that represents feeling calm, like your true self, and ready for whatever comes next. Also decide what number(s) mean a no-go as far as starting your session.

Really take a minute to think about whether you are in a state of too high or too low arousal to really be an effective CP. Always remember that the regulation required as a CP is just as important (if not more so) than your ability to prompt and switch boards.

Next, assess your speller's readiness to do a session right now. If it seems like they aren't ready yet, consider doing some intentional motor exercises as a warm up. This can help bring low arousal levels up as well as high arousal levels down. You might also start by reading together or doing a short breathing meditation together. Extending the outbreath in particular is what helps to activate the parasympathetic nervous system and lower arousal levels to the just-right regulation state. You might also try a guided visualization activity together before starting your session, or even play some soft classical music in the background.

Another key ingredient to a successfully coregulated session is to not lose sight of the fact that apraxia is a brain-body disconnect. Whatever "behavior" your speller is exhibiting, and behavior simply means something they're doing with their body, it may not be reflective of how they're truly feeling on the inside. It also may not be purposeful. As parents, it can be hard to stay regulated when our child appears to be "acting out" or "misbehaving" but for the exclusive time that they are spelling with you we recommend setting aside any preconceived beliefs. Just for the twenty to thirty minutes of your session, act purely as a partner and a motor coach. If they lie face down on the floor, avoid parenting their behavior. Tell yourself "this is just a motor problem with impulsivity" and coach their body back to the chair. If they repeatedly script "all done!" continue taking your own deep breaths and calmly remind them that you're planning to spend this twenty-minute commitment with them no matter what. Explain that you'll just read for the next few minutes while they get their body more settled.

If you don't make spelling the actual goal of your session with your child, you'll ironically have much greater success in the long run. If you make connecting with your child the goal of the session, then you will keep strengthening the bond between you. Focusing on regulation in a session may ultimately result in them poking some letters on a stencil, or it may simply result in you snuggling together while you read the lesson out loud and trace words with your finger into the palm of their hand. Either way, the core of any successful speller-CP dyad is the strength of the connection between the two people involved.

Many times, we have seen there is PTSD or shared trauma in the families where spellers have a history of injurious or self-injurious behavior. This history does make it difficult for parents to lean into any dysregulation that their child begins to feel, and understandably so. That's another great reason to make connection the goal first and foremost. A relationship that has been through trauma together would certainly benefit from shared tender moments on this path toward letterboard fluency. Take your time with this entire process and rekindle the interbrain connection you had at the time of their birth.

We can't stress enough how healing it might also be for parents to work with a family therapist and even consider some trauma release work if appropriate. In fact, once your speller gains some fluency, they might also appreciate such therapy for themselves as well. At the start of the spelled communication journey, everyone sets their sights on achieving open communication and rightfully so. But we'd like to offer you the idea that open communication is just the first significant milestone on a whole new recalibration process. Once fluent, there will also be things to unpack together as a family to achieve the health, happiness, and healing that all of you deserve.

DYSREGULATION

If you opened this handbook and started here first, we feel you. We wish we could provide a perfect blueprint for consistently peaceful spelling sessions, but the truth is—learning Spellers Method is hard work. At times it's not going to be easy, in fact, sometimes it can be downright messy, but it will always be worth it. With that said, there are many things we do in sessions to help avoid dysregulation or de-escalate it when it first begins. The timing of interventions to help a speller stay regulated is especially important.

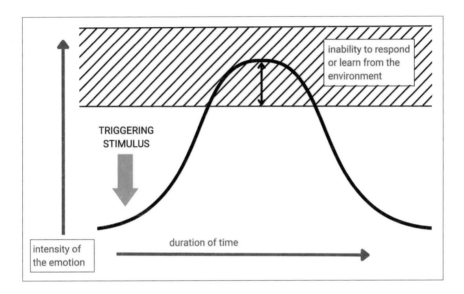

Let's start by defining dysregulation. It is the state in which a person is unable to control or "regulate" their own emotional or physical response to stimuli around them. It may also be described as a dramatic fluctuation in mood or emotions resulting in anger outbursts, injurious actions toward oneself or others, or other damaging behaviors. As you can see from the simple diagram above, once the intensity of a person's emotion goes up their ability to respond to or learn from the environment around them also decreases. De-escalating a speller before they hit the "red zone" is ideal whenever possible.

As stated in the previous section on coregulation, when a person is dysregulated, they are *not* using the cortical part of their brain to think. Have you ever seen T-shirts that say "All behavior is communication?" Well, that actually isn't true. A lot of behavior is an involuntary reaction to a perceived threat, a threat that may not even be universally scary. For example, many people respond in fight, flight, or freeze when they see a spider in the bathroom, while others gently cup the critter in their bare hands and release it outside to freedom. The spider example goes to show you that the stimulus is actually neutral, but the perceived threat poses a real problem to someone's ability to regulate themselves. Furthermore, telling someone afraid of spiders to "calm down" has never, in the history of mankind, helped the arachnophobic person chill out.

This concept of perceived threat is important so that we learn to respect our child's unique experience of the world, even when we don't fully understand it ourselves. Insisting a child "get over it" or telling them "You're fine!" is actually a form of gaslighting. Though it might be our innocent and feeble attempt at coregulation, in your child's immediate experience of dysregulation, they're *anything but* fine. Instead, we try to say things like "You're safe" or "You're going to be okay." Telling someone who's freaking out that they're already fine is, well, triggering! If they could speak, they'd probably scream back "I am *not* fine!" But without speech, they just end up escalating more. So, let's not add kerosene to the fire, shall we?

Seeing them as dysregulated and acknowledging they are dysregulated can be very helpful to the student. Here are examples of some things you can softly say:

> I see you're upset.
> I can see your body is dysregulated.
> Let's pause... hold your body...
> You're safe. Everything will be okay. (Which is different than saying "You're okay!")

In the case of dysregulation during a spelling session, the student's actions are rarely the result of conscious choices. Their muscles and resulting behaviors are occurring from impulses sent by the amygdala and brain stem. Quite literally, their nervous system is doing everything it can to escape the lion. Oftentimes it's best not to speak at all but rather to begin modeling calming strategies yourself. Ground your own energy, take slow deep breaths and extend those outbreaths for at least a count of four, give the spellers some space. As a way to prevent dysregulation, you might start this practice before you even invite your child to come practice spelling with you.

We understand that your child might have a repertoire of behavior that prior therapists have labeled as "escape" or "task avoidance." We also know that spellers are human beings and sure, they might not always want to do what we are asking them to do. *But* in the case of having a successful spelling session, this is where the principles of presuming competence paired with coaching the motor go hand in hand.

Remember first the least dangerous assumption. That is the belief that your child can and does want to learn, that they can and do want to participate in the spelling session; however, their nervous system is misinterpreting stimuli and is responding in fight or flight. Using logical persuasion to de-escalate your child is rarely effective. Instead, if you can separate in your mind your old ideas about what they're behavior means and trust us that their behavior is simply the result of their faulty neuroception, you'll be in a much better place to support their regulation successfully. This is step one to avoiding dysregulation: checking your own beliefs and setting aside the ones that don't empower you to be a strong coregulation partner.

Step two is to put the oxygen mask on yourself. A rule of thumb we often suggest is that when you notice your speller's arousal level going up, you should adjust your affect and energy down. Slow your body movements, speak in a softer voice, and pause between statements if you speak at all. This is one of the best early interventions to potential dysregulation.

Now let's just play devil's advocate and say they really don't want to spell right now. We can't know this for sure, but for the sake of argument let's presume it's the case. What do you do in that situation? This is why we recommend deciding in advance how much time you're committing to spelling with your child that day. Rather than "playing it by ear" which usually means quitting the session as soon as they get dysregulated or not even starting if they greet you with "no, no, no, no," you'll be committed to finding tools in your toolbox to coregulate, at least until your timer goes off. This is so important for building your own confidence as a regulation partner and also for building their confidence in being able to do hard things! It's the ultimate resiliency builder.

Refer back to the section on the motor and cognitive continuums. Learning to adjust the motor or cognitive demand is a very effective way to work through that. If the dysregulation starts at the beginning of the session, then your best approach is to engage in some intentional motor exercises as a warm-up instead. You can find a series of helpful videos modeling different intentional motor exercises here.

Intentional Motor

TOP-DOWN VERSUS BOTTOM-UP REGULATION

When we are coaching parents to help coregulate during a spelling session or anytime their child is dysregulated, we typically talk about doing so in two ways—top-down or bottom-up regulation. Let's discuss the two approaches and learn how the solution is not always one or the other, but can also be a combination of the two.

Bottom-up regulation is when we are using sensory-based strategies to help to calm your speller. When our spellers experience flight or fight and the lower brain centers are triggered, they need support to calm so that they can get back to utilizing their "thinking" brain. We, as non-apraxic individuals, are able to get back from fight or flight with greater ease. If you think about how we do that, it is often more from a bottom-up approach to regulation. For example, when stressed, we may go for a walk which is rhythmic, activates the proprioceptors, and regulates breathing. Others may head to the gym or go for a run. Bottom-up regulation and what works is very individualized. For spellers when working in a spelling session, there are a number of ways that we can implement a bottom-up approach to regulation. For example, speaking in a softer voice, perhaps using some rhythm and counting while we are giving some deep pressure, or starting out the session with some intentional movement in the gym. All of these strategies help calm the nervous system so that we can get the body in a place where they can move more intentionally and get back to spelling.

Another approach to regulation is via top-down strategies. The reason it's called "top-down" is because we are targeting the "higher thinking" areas of the brain. These are cognitive-based strategies that require the speller to think and process what they are hearing. This is one of the reasons why we use age appropriate lessons. It's a top-down strategy to regulation. Top-down regulation is also very individualized and there are spellers who need extra cognitive input in addition to a lesson. Examples include listening to podcasts, college lectures, audiobooks, or TED Talks. These can be playing on your phone or computer at very low volume while doing a lesson. Sometimes spellers prefer to wear headphones while listening and others are okay with it on the phone or computer.

> **Dana:** As an OT top-down regulation as a strategy for individuals with autism was never something that was taught. OT's were very focused on sensory-based strategies mainly because I was taught that those with non-speaking autism and unreliably speaking individuals have an intellectual delay so why would I consider top-down regulation for a strategy? Well, low and behold it works! After learning from spellers over the years some of them need such high cognitive input to support regulation it blows my mind. I have multiple spellers who wear

Bluetooth headphones with a Harvard lecture playing while they are doing a lesson with me. Other spellers benefit from lessons in a different language because it's cognitively challenging. I now never underestimate the power of high-level cognitive input for my spellers!

Top-down and bottom-up strategies to regulation can and are often used simultaneously. For example, during a spelling session a speller may need additional cognitive input which is playing in his headphones and he may need some proprioceptive input and rhythm to get his body in a place for spelling. Spellers Method practitioners are trained to coach parents on what their child needs specifically for regulation. It's important to have a conversation and ask questions so you know how to support your child during their session for success.

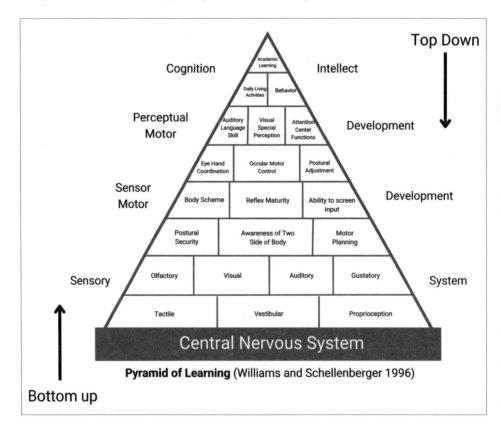

Pyramid of Learning (Williams and Schellenberger 1996)

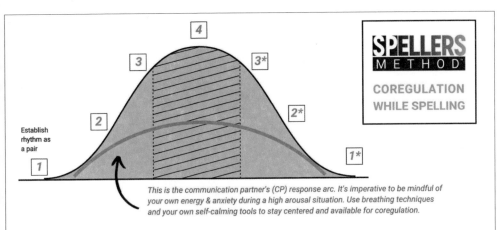

This is the communication partner's (CP) response arc. It's imperative to be mindful of your own energy & anxiety during a high arousal situation. Use breathing techniques and your own self-calming tools to stay centered and available for coregulation.

1 Find your groove together. Proactively employ bottom up sensory strategies as a warm up, then move straight into your spelling session. Create a rhythm together from first contact.

2 At first sign of early stress, focus the student's attention away from it. Use the motor-cognitive balance to adjust demand and maintain regulation on the boards; offer body engagers.

3 Engage their body more fully in intentional motor exercises and/or calming strategies. Do not ask student to make choices. Coach their body with clear, simple instructions. Model deep breaths.

4 This is peak anxiety time for the student and may include injurious behavior towards self/others. Avoid speaking if possible. Use gestures, move slowly, model calming strategies. Don't rush this moment.

3* Using slow speech and encouraging words, gently woo your student back into intentional motor OR start reading the lesson content (top-down regulation strategy) without asking them to spell yet.

2* Continue to model calming techniques, engage student in spelling again, and regain rhythm and flow on the boards. Continue to offer body engagers.

1* The strength of a relationship isn't based on never having a breakdown; it's in what happens after the breakdown and repair. Celebrate your successful co-navigation of a high arousal situation & give positive feedback to the student on what they did well today. Give yourself some credit too!

(c) 2023 Spellers Revolution

16

So, Now What?
Life After You Embark

It can be challenging to learn something new, and learning to spell with your son or daughter can be one of those times. We've all been in a position where we feel vulnerable, and it takes courage and a willingness to jump into uncharted territory to proceed. We know that *all* parents can become their child's communication partner. We are not suggesting that it's easy, breezy, but you can do it! Working with a Spellers Method practitioner will ensure you have the support and guidance you need to build your confidence as a CP. We work with CPs that have learning disabilities and those that have anxiety or PTSD. We can work alongside you to find the best way for you to embody the best CP for your speller. Besides taking a deep breath and jumping right in, here are a few other tips to help ease your mind.

1. The first time you spell with your son or daughter can be nerve-racking but don't fear! It's normal to be embarrassed because suddenly you can't remember the

word you're spelling or the next letter in the word *fire*! You, too, are learning a new motor skill and trying to balance the motor and cognitive demands of being a CP. You're also working hard to regulate yourself *and* regulate your child. Don't be too hard on yourself. Like any new motor skill, you have learned, this will become automatic with time.

2. While working hard to be a CP for your child, you're also trying to help regulate them. You may find that your typical regulation support involved "feathering their nest." It's a process for us all to avoid falling into our automatic responses. Still, it's essential to focus on the lesson and remember that it will be easier if you coach their motor skills (spelling) and not worry about their seemingly unmet physical needs. If your child is an unreliable speaker and repeats a phrase or words continuously, respond once and then continue with the lesson. Remember, we are presuming competence, so we believe your child fully understands when you say, "We will get lunch right after our lesson." So if they ask about lunch every three minutes, continue to coach their body to spell. This is most likely a motor loop that spelling can break. This, too, will get easier!

3. We discussed prompting and prompt dependency earlier, but reiterating here is essential. Depending on your therapy experience, you may believe your child will become prompt dependent if you prompt too much. We are all "prompt dependent" to a certain degree. With respect to apraxia, one of the most challenging things to do is to initiate a movement. When the speller starts spelling, we use strong initiation prompts, strong gestural prompts for the eyes, and strong directional prompts. If we think about it, initiation is involved in every movement the speller makes. We encourage CPs

to over-prompt because one of the initial goals is to build a solid rhythm and pace. If you are holding back on your prompts, this can become difficult because your speller may not be able to get their eyes to the top corner "A," and they begin to miss-poke. That may dysregulate them, which may dysregulate you, and then the rhythm and pace are disrupted. As you are building your skills, don't be afraid to over-prompt. We promise you, spellers become independent of our prompts.

4. Stick with it till the end. What we mean by that is support your speller to finish the last word rather than ending halfway through the word because they are dysregulated or their body can't sit in the chair. Finishing up the word and supporting the speller as much as possible to finish is one of the strongest ways to build your relationship. Nothing says, "I'm here with you no matter what," more than finishing the last word of the lesson when the speller is having a difficult time with their body. Your practitioner can help guide you on the best way to work through this with your specific speller.

5. Avoid "keeping up with the Joneses." This is one of the most challenging things for families. They see a speller, even a speller similar to their child's profile, and it seems their child is struggling more. Quick thoughts can take over: "Maybe he can't do this," "Am I pushing something that shouldn't happen?" or "What am I doing wrong as his CP?" All of these questions are ones that families have asked us about before. The truth is, every speller is different. It's tough to compare any one speller's trajectory on the letterboards to another's. What *is* important is to reach out to your practitioner if you are feeling discouraged. We are happy to talk with you! Remember, your family's journey is your family's journey. Each speller's journey is different. Enjoy your

time together (yes, we realize not all spelling sessions will be joyous, but try!) as you build your skills on the boards.

WHAT WILL THIS COST YOU?

1. **Time**—We suggest daily practice. Sometimes that isn't doable for a family, so practice as many days each week as possible. That may be two or three times per week, but that is better than not starting at all! Remind yourself that you and your child are learning a new motor skill. No professional athlete can become proficient or compete in the Olympics with just three months of practice. It took hard work, dedication, and daily practice. The same goes for learning the motor skill of spelling. Go for the gold!

2. **Money**—What price is too high to hear your child's authentic voice? Yes, learning the Spellers Method will be an investment in the beginning as you are working with a practitioner. However, this is a parent-driven program, and it all boils down to the practice you do between your sessions with a practitioner. It's essential to look at this differently than typical therapy such as OT or speech therapy. Your practitioner may also be one of those clinicians, but spelling is meant to be something you participate in both in the session and at home.

3. **Reorganized Priorities**—No one ever said that life would always feel fair, and generation after generation of siblings have fought over perceived slights in their

family's hierarchy of needs at one time or another. It is important to recognize your family unit as an entire system. Sort of like an ecosystem; each part is dependent on and affected by the whole. Sometimes, one part of the system needs a lot of attention while the other parts need to adjust to having less. Then things change, as they always do, and resources become allocated back to those that got by with less for a while. Getting comfortable with the inequality of resource division (i.e., your time and attention) as you embark on your spelling journey is a necessary step. You will need to dedicate enough time and attention to your speller during the acquisition phase of the Spellers Method so they can make steady progress. Just remember, this is a massive investment in the entire family, not just your nonspeaker, and it will all be worth it.

4. **Facing Any Guilt**—This is a challenging one for many parents. There are moments when parents first realize that their child *does* understand all that's being said around them, and the parents feel an incredible amount of guilt knowing some of the things that they have said in front of their child before. Everyone has a set of beliefs that drive their decisions and what they say. At that time, you had the belief that your child did not understand what you were saying. It's okay. Forgive yourself. This may take some time to process, and that is okay too. *You* are your child's greatest resource. Letting go of any guilt or shame from the past is essential for the healthy development of your relationship with your CP-speller.

5. **Falling in Love with Not Knowing**—You've now discovered spelled communication and everything you previously thought about your child might have been wrong. Not only do you realize your nonspeaker has

always been comprehending the world around them, but they're also highly intelligent and full of the same hopes, dreams, feelings, and ideas a neurotypical child would have. This shift into a new way of life can be tricky for parents, siblings, and other caregivers to navigate. There is no manual on how to adjust both your mindset and your practical approach in helping to support that same child from now on. Your speller now has the agency to plan a self-directed life of passion and purpose, yet they might also require a lot of physical support to achieve their dreams. Be patient with yourself and this process as you adjust to new roles. Be open to admitting when you are wrong and ask your speller to guide you on what they need from you. This can be uncomfortable at first, but at the end of the day, it's also entirely liberating for everyone involved. Ask other parents who've traveled this road before you for suggestions on how to let go and empower your speller to have more and more agency.

WHY DO WE RECOMMEND WORKING WITH A PRACTITIONER?

1. **They Can Help Break Down Motor Coaching into Easy, Straightforward Steps.** The first session with a practitioner can make spelling look "easy." However, sitting down beside your child to start your first spelling session can bring anxiety and nerves front and center! Suddenly you forget how to spell the word *Construction* because you're thinking of a million things simultaneously! This is totally normal but also highlights the

importance of working with a Spellers Method practitioner to give you a solid start. We have worked with many families who have attempted to start on their own without any support, and they fully admit that it was challenging and, at the time, did not think their child was a "good fit" for spelling because they "couldn't do it." Spelling is a shift in the paradigm that you have been told for the last however many years—your child has an intellectual disability, your child will only reach the cognitive capacity of a six-month-old, or your child has an IQ of forty. This mindset shift can take time. It's easy to go back into this thinking when your child pokes the wrong letter or doesn't initiate poking it. When you work with a practitioner, they can support your progress and remind you that this is a motor disability and coach you through any plateaus that you may experience.

2. **They Can Empower You with Confidence as the Leader of Your Child's Communication Journey.** Confidence is one of the most critical components of the parent/speller relationship. Any CP working with a speller must be confident, and Spellers Method practitioners have many tools to help you gain the confidence to spell with your child. We have coached hundreds of CPs. Some have learning disabilities, and others struggle to gain confidence, but we have not worked with any CP that could not build the skills needed to spell. Just like our spellers, some CPs have a more prolonged acquisition phase when learning the skills. We recommend that CPs contact a practitioner when they need support or if something isn't going well. Don't quit! We will empower you with the skills you need to continue to spell together.

3. **They Will Never Give Up on You or Your Speller.** Never will we give up! All of our families can learn

Spellers Method. Each family is a unique system of beliefs, emotions, and experiences that are brought to the table. Our practitioners are trained to support you where you need it most and know how to support you in each moment, even when you may want to give up. Your speller may have more motor complexities that may make the acquisition phase of spelling longer, and that's okay! This is about hearing your child's authentic voice. We have worked with families who repeatedly ask us if "we are sure this is the right method for their child." We always say "Yes" because Spellers Method practitioners understand your child's motor complexities and sensory-motor differences. We will never give up on you or your child!

4. **They Will Support You in a Nonjudgmental, Collaborative Way.** Spellers Method practitioners have worked with many families and coached hundreds of communication partners to support their spellers' reliable communication. We value family and building relationships and understand that families come from different backgrounds and experiences. We know that as parents, you are doing your very best for your child, and we are here for one thing—to support your family no matter what. This is a parent/caregiver–driven program and requires time and commitment each day. We get that life happens, and things come up unexpectedly, which is okay! We will meet you where you are and come alongside you so that you can be confident in your abilities to support your child.

5. **They Will Guide You through a Paradigm-Shifting Experience That Will Forever Change How You View Your Child and Your Future Together.** As practitioners, this is one of our favorite things! We get to see the change in each family that we work with. It's amazing to see

the shift in parents as they start to presume competence in their child. We often hear comments such as, "Once I realized that they do understand what I am saying, even though they may not look like they are listening, they (the child) seemed more confident and happier!" When families can shift and disregard what they have been told about their child's abilities, both physically and cognitively, the entire family dynamics change. One of our families said, "Each day comes with its challenges because our son is still apraxic and struggles to control his body, but knowing that he understands it all and wants to gain control of his body completely changes our mindset. We have so much joy!"

17

So, What's Next?

You made it to the end of the handbook! Congratulations. Some of you may now be wondering, what's next?

The answer is simply: *practice, practice, and more practice*! Once you've had an assessment done, whether in person or online, with a trained Spellers Method practitioner, they will give you specific things to work on at home. Daily practice is the goal, but we understand that life happens. Schedules change, and all of us have tough days. Don't sweat it. Even if there's been some time off between practice sessions, just pick up where you left off in the previous session and keep moving forward. As the saying goes, this isn't a sprint but a marathon. Just like the fans cheering runners from the sidelines, we are here to cheer you on. When you encounter a problem, it's essential to contact your practitioner and ask questions as soon as possible. If you ever find that you are at a plateau or wondering what the next step is, consider that an excellent time to schedule another session or two with your practitioner. Our goal is to coach you and your speller to the next level so you can keep moving forward.

So what happens when—Bam!—Some emotions surface that need processing?

Don't be alarmed if this happens to you, it's normal. Working through buried emotions (yours and your speller's) after you start spelling can be immediate for some and take time for others. Some folks never experience an emotional upheaval, aside from bliss, that is. Everyone's experience is different. But over the years, as we worked with families, we've been asked many questions. This is all part of the process. Here are a few common ones, though the true list goes on and on:

- *Why hasn't anyone told me about spelled communication sooner?* We often hear this and know it's a significant issue—most people aren't even aware that individuals with apraxia *can* communicate. This can bring up some resentment, anger, and even guilt for somehow not knowing (even though no one told you). Our best suggestion is to allow yourself those feelings and feel them big, but set a time limit to it. Give yourself a day, or maybe a week, to be mad, feel guilty, you name it. But when the time expires, let those feelings go and move on to the present moment. Don't keep looking backwards. You're not going that way! The future *is* bright and you don't want to hinder your forward momentum with emotions over things in the past that can't be changed.
- *How do I handle my speller's feelings and the dysregulation that sometimes accompanies finally being able to express those pent-up emotions?* We know you've waited a long time for this moment; however, we strongly advise not barreling into the decade-long list of things you "always wanted to know" about your child as soon as they become an open speller. Achieving open

communication for the first time after years of silence is a *lot* for anyone to process. New spellers often aren't equipped to handle the flood of emotions that comes with highly emotional topics right away. Not to mention, it's kind of nice to let them tell us what they've been dying to say first.

- As for those things you want to know, we typically suggest doing structured lessons on those topics and working your open questions into the text instead. A trained practitioner can guide you through this. Once your speller has had more time spelling openly on the boards, it typically won't be as overwhelming to ask a personal question on an emotional topic. In the meantime, we advise just taking it slow and easy. Let your speller bring up the topics they want first.

- ***How does this new revelation of your nonspeaking child's intact intelligence and understanding of the world around them impact their siblings?*** Our biggest suggestion for you regarding how this impacts the rest of the family is to find outside resources to support you in this new chapter of your journey together. Marriage and family therapists as well as counselors are often key resources to help unpack all the things that come to the surface. The family is a system, and the whole is greater than the sum of its parts. That means that the relationships between each member are intricate, interrelated, and impact the whole. Spelling affects everyone! Your Spellers Method practitioner may be able to share some anecdotes from families who've walked the road before you, but anything beyond that is outside their scope of practice—unless they are licensed therapists themselves. Countless families have chosen to pursue outside help to navigate their new journey together. We highly recommend you consider the same!

Meanwhile, we would love to leave you with a few parting suggestions. These are meant to help you navigate the acquisition phase of spelling with greater success and enjoyment.

- Understand that relationships grow potential. Connect with your child during spelling sessions *first* and *foremost*. Make the actual spelling the secondary goal during sessions.
- Celebrate learning alongside your speller. Give yourself permission to be vulnerable, to make mistakes, and to forge this new path together as partners.
- Forget that you're a parent while on the letterboard. Just be their CP. It will make your decision-making algorithm much simpler: just coach their motor.
- Always remember to put the oxygen mask on yourself first during any moment of dysregulation. It's the best way to help yourself and your speller get through it and be a stronger dyad as a result.
- Know that progress is rarely linear for any new speller. Occasional back steps or side steps are part of the process. Don't panic, just stay the course. With guidance from a practitioner you will find your way back to forward momentum.
- Don't go it alone, even if you live far away from any trained practitioners or other spelling families. Get connected in our online Spellers Community on Facebook. There are hundreds of families with years of spelling practice under their belt wanting to pay it forward with their experience and hope. Get plugged in and share your own highs and lows with your fellow families.

18

Advice from Fluent Spellers to Your Nonspeaker

Lora: What to Expect When You're Spelling

When my mom was pregnant, she had a book called *What to Expect When You're Expecting*. That book was her bible while she awaited the birth of each of her five daughters. I wanted to help my fellow spellers know what to expect when spelling. I hope my experience will help guide your spelling journey.

First, you will notice that not everyone believes you are capable of learning to communicate. Your teachers or even some family members might be skeptical because they have seen you as intellectually disabled for years. When you start to spell for the first time, they will say you don't know what you're doing because you will have a hard time making your body poke the letters your brain is telling it to. That's OK. Whatever you do, don't give up!

With months of practice, you will show the haters they were wrong.

Next, don't forget to tell yourself that the spelling journey will bring out emotions that have been buried inside you for years. At first you will feel nervous and apprehensive because no one before has assumed you have the prose and poetry in you that has always been present in your soul and brain. Try to understand that they have been doing the best they can based on what the childhood developmental "experts" have told them. Really try to forgive them so you can move forward.

Don't forget to go there in terms of seeing all the possibilities in front of you now that you can communicate. There are so many things to decide. What will you do with your new voice? How will you help free other non-speakers? Very soon there will be a revolution and you are a warrior on the front lines. Be prepared to do your part to win the war. The enemy is heavily armed.

Forge ahead in life. When you hit a wall, remember you will bounce back. There will be times when you are discouraged and hopeless. Stay on the path and pay attention to the politics that work against us. You are not alone. Have faith in your abilities, and when you feel like giving up, think of all the future spellers you are helping to liberate from their silent prisons.

There will be an earthly army of spiteful, angry people that will try to tell the world that we are not committed to our cause. They will say that we are not the ones communicating. You must try to ignore them if we are to triumph. When our numbers soar, we can bring the truth to light.

by Lora Tompkins (age 18, Las Vegas, Nevada)

Amelia: Dear New Speller

The need to be seen and to feel known is shared by many. For most nonspeakers, being unseen is a devastating reality. In the years before I learned to communicate by spelling, the frustration of being misunderstood was a constant, and despair threatened to overcome me. Those closest to me believed that my favorite color was pink, that I loved the food from a particular fast food chicken restaurant, and that coloring books were my preferred activity, when in fact I dislike all of those things. More significantly, there was a firm belief about my intellectual ability that dictated an educational program that was mind numbing. In the months immediately prior to spelling, as I approached my 13th birthday, I spent my days "learning" single digit addition and reading from picture books. The low expectations also extended to my emotional capabilities, leading to the cruel assumption that I could not comprehend things like empathy or love, much less form friendships or romantic relationships. In countless meetings with experts, misconceptions about me were repeated as facts as if I was not present, and I could do nothing to alter the perceptions that shaped my life.

Communication has the potential to change nearly every aspect of your life, because it is the means by which you can finally let others begin to see the person that you are and have always been. In the three years since I started spelling, more has shifted than I would have dared to expect. Last year I was admitted to a competitive public collegiate high school and I finished my junior year with a 4.0 grade point average. College-level textbooks and real works of fiction and nonfiction have replaced picture books, and I can now discuss those books with friends and "neurotypical" classmates. Writing poetry has become a great source of peace, and I have felt the joy of having my poems published, set to music and performed publicly. I have also experienced the thrill of my first romantic relationship with a wonderful fellow speller, along with the difficult process of a breakup. My relationships with family members are now filled with shared insights and decision-making. Among the most consequential changes is what I have gained through deep friendships with other nonspeakers. In meetings in-person and online, through their words and through their presence, they are an unwavering source of strength, support and understanding.

If you or your family are reading this, I hope that means that you are on or near the path of being able to openly communicate. Whatever it takes, please keep pushing until you are able to share some of your true self with the world. When you are ready, we will be here waiting to see you, yearning to know you.

Amelia Bell

Elliot Sylvester: A Letter to New Spellers
As a walking advertisement for how spelling can change your life, it is my pleasure to share these words of inspiration with you now. Future spellers, life ahead is full of a light unlike you have experienced. Using a letterboard to communicate opens doors that have been long closed to unreliable speakers and nonspeakers alike. Now is our time to arise and step into a life well lived. I am asking for spellers new and well-practiced to join our family. The revolution awaits you. Start this journey knowing that it will be hard work but so worth it.

Sincerely,
Elliot

Hunter Oliver: To Parents of Future Spellers

Don't underestimate your child. They are very competent and intelligent but have no way of showing you who they truly are without a way to communicate. Spelling has changed my life in a way that is hard to describe. Through spelling I am able to express myself on a deeper level than speech would ever allow me. Please give your child the opportunity to become the person they are capable of.

Sincerely,
Hunter

Abigail Gore: Dear Future Speller and Family

I want so much to tell you how spelling has changed my life. I am a nonspeaker with autism and Downs and before I spelled to communicate, I was viewed as an unintelligent person with no potential. However, now I have found my voice and I have so much to say to the world about presuming competence in those who have limited speech and disabilities. Give us the opportunity to learn and you will quickly find out how much we have to offer society. Your child is capable of endless things if given the chance and the proper support. Starting can be challenging and there will be ups and downs but anything worth achieving requires hard work and I have faith in you.

Sincerely,
Abigail

Austin Keefer: Dear New Speller and Their Support

As my letter finds you, anything about nonspeakers that you thought you knew is going to change drastically. At this time neurodiverse people are on a long road to accessing communication by all of the ways we can spell.

From my own ongoing journey, I can tell you that it is more work than it sounds but the reward is all worth it. As I think back to when I started spelling, I shared a skepticism with my parents. I had no idea the impact that it would have on my life. As I began communicating my thoughts and started going to a school that treated me with the respect I deserved, my life became more fulfilling than I could have imagined. Almost five years later, I am on a path to college and all of that is in connection to my family's commitment to me learning to spell. Rarely do I say this, but nothing is more important than my ability to communicate with others.

Shared from the heart,
Austin Keefer

Jack Maynard

I would like to address the parents of a nonspeaking individual—I want to say please believe in your child. I promise you that they are capable of learning to spell their thoughts, feelings, and knowledge and all they need is practice and your support. I know the beginning will be tough because we suffer from motor apraxia but trust me, it will be life changing for not only your child but your entire family. If you need further proof, please come visit us at Excel26 so you can meet me and my friends. You will be able to hear about our personal journeys on learning to spell to communicate and your doubts will wash away.

With love,
Jack Maynard

Macrae Chittum: A Letter to New Spellers and Their Families:

You are about to embark on the greatest experience of your life. Spelling can offer you a lifelong ability to communicate your thoughts reliably. In time the words will flow freely and unlock your potential to have a meaningful existence in this crazy world. As communication becomes more and more reliable, frustration over being misunderstood will just melt away and you will have a sense of peace for the first time in your life. Don't second guess yourself and be confident in your ability while you practice. Take advantage of every opportunity to spell because practice is the key to success. This will be life changing and open doors previously thought to be welded shut. I'm not even exaggerating about the huge impact spelling to communicate will have on your quality of life. It's undeniable. Parents—don't underestimate your child and be sure to presume competence. We are always listening and taking it all in, so we know more than you think and need your support during the process. Lean on fellow spellers and their families and be sure to reach out if you need anything. Our community is strong, and we support each other without judgment. It makes me smile to think of the bright future that will be revealed using Spelling. In letters we trust!

Stay strong,
Macrae Chittum

Glossary of Terms

AAC	Augmentative and Alternative Communication covers all the ways that a person can communicate besides talking. This includes methods such as speech generating devices (an app on a tablet, iPad, or computer), pointing to pictures or symbols, using choice cards, spelling for communication, RPM (rapid prompting method), sign language, gestures, and even facial expressions.
Ableism	Ableism is a form of social prejudice that favors able-bodied people and discriminates against those with disabilities. Attempting to make an autistic person appear or behave like a neurotypical person is an example of ableism.
Acquisition phase	The acquisition phase, also known as the "skill building" phase, occurs anytime the speller is acquiring the motor skills to accurately point at letters on the letterboard to build fluency. Spellers are in the application phase when they first begin spelling and again each time they move up the motor continuum to a new board with a higher motor demand. An example of this is moving from the three boards to the 26 board or from the laminate board to the keyboard.
Amygdala	The amygdala is an almond-shaped region of the brain primarily associated with emotional processes. It impacts the way a person experiences cognition, exhibits emotional learning, handles social interaction, and processes social input.

Application phase	A speller enters the application phase when they are able to reliably use the letterboard skills learned in the acquisition phase to communicate openly in the community. For example: using a 26 board to order at a restaurant, create goals for school, or join the boy scouts. A speller can be in both the acquisition and application phase at the same while progressing up the motor continuum, e.g., fluently spelling on the laminate board while acquiring the skills to do known questions on the keyboard.
Apraxia	Apraxia is a condition where an individual can't complete the steps of intentional motor planning due to a neurological difference even though they can understand what is being asked of them. Other terms often used in place of apraxia include: *dyspraxia, developmental coordination disorder (DCD), sensory integration disorder, sensory processing disorder, motor planning differences, fine motor delay, gross motor delay, behavioral disorder,* etc. What's most important to remember is that apraxia is not a sign of cognitive impairment.
Arcuate fasciculus	A bundle of fibers in the brain that connects the temporal lobe to the frontal lobe. One of its key responsibilities is connecting Broca's and Wernicke's areas, which are the areas in the brain responsible for producing and understanding language.
Arousal level	Arousal level refers to the physiological state of being alert, attentive, non-distracted, and aware of the situation. Arousal level can be mental, physical, and emotional. It impacts a person's ability to effectively perform any task on demand with efficiency.

Assistive technology	Assistive technology (AT) is any item, piece of equipment, software program, or product system whether acquired commercially off the shelf, modified, or customized that is used to increase, maintain, or improve the functional capabilities of persons with disabilities. The term does not include a medical device that is surgically implanted, or the replacement of such device. https://sites.ed.gov/idea/regs/b/a/300.5
Assistive technology device (examples)	Assistive technology devices include both high-tech and low-tech communication devices such as: letter boards for spelled communication, PECS, Ipads, speech generating devices, and other communication assisted technology. AT devices can also be hardware such as prosthetics, mounting systems, and positioning devices. It can include computer software such as screen readers and communication programs. It can be inclusive or specialized learning materials, curriculum aids, eye gaze and head trackers. It can also be mobility devices such as wheelchairs, walkers, braces, power lifts, and more.
Assistive technology service	An assistive technology service means any service that directly assists a child with a disability in the selection, acquisition, or use of an assistive technology device. https://sites.ed.gov/idea/statute-chapter-33/subchapter-i/1401
Bloom's taxonomy	Bloom's taxonomy is a hierarchical model used in education. It scaffolds increasingly more complex levels of cognition in the areas of thinking, learning, and understanding.

Body engagers	An activity that requires intentional motor (usually involving the hands) to help engage, still, and regulate a speller's body while listening or learning. Examples of body engagers include: sticker puzzle books, a word search, beading a necklace, or cutting or traces images. *Body engagers are different from "fidgets" which do not require any intentional motor to complete, e.g., a pop it or fidget spinner.
Bottom-Up regulation	Bottom-up regulation involves using sensory-based strategies to help calm your speller and return them to a learner-ready state of arousal. When a speller experiences fight or flight and the sympathetic nervous system is activated, deep breathing exercises, deep proprioceptive input to the muscles, intentional motor activities, and even lowering the head below the heart are all examples of bottom-up strategies to return the nervous system into a parasympathetic state and bring awareness back to their "thinking" brain.
Brainstem	The brainstem is the lower part of the brain that connects it to the spinal cord. It is responsible for controlling all the automatic features of the body including breathing, blood pressure, heart rate, and sleep.
Broca's area	A region of the brain located in the cerebral cortex that is primarily associated with language production. This area plays a role in the ability to sequence words together effectively to create sentences, thoughts, and ideas in an articulate manner.
Caudate nucleus	C-shaped subcortical structure which lies deep inside the brain near the thalamus. It plays a critical role in various higher neurological functions.

Continuation prompt	Continuation prompts are steady and continuous verbal prompts used to keep a speller's motor going. These prompts are said rhythmically by the communication partner in between letters of a word or a sentence. The speller's motor hooks onto the voice of the CP which helps to sustain the speller's motor. Words that can be used as continuation prompts include: and, then, next letter is, keep moving, and travel.
Convergence insufficiency	Convergence insufficiency is an eye condition that impacts how your eyes work together as a team when you attempt to look at nearby objects, like a letterboard.
Core words	Core words, or core vocabulary, are terms used to describe a relatively small set of words that are used most frequently in oral and written language. It has been estimated that on average we use the same four hundred words for about 80 percent of our daily communication.
Cortical brain	The cortical brain, or cerebral cortex, refers to four lobes of the brain. It is sometimes referred to as the "thinking" brain. These regions deal with different modalities of sensation, often relayed by the spinal cord or directly by the cranial nerves. Moreover, one of these regions initiates conscious motor movement.
CP	CP is an acronym for communication partner. When spelling with a nonspeaker, you take on the role as their CP. Think of this as being a coregulator to help assist in maintaining the speller's regulation, while also being a motor coach to assist them in executing the motor sequences to communicate through spelling.
Cranial nerves	The cranial nerves are a set of twelve paired nerves that come from the back of your brain. They send electrical signals between your brain, face, neck, and torso. These nerves help you taste, smell, hear, and feel sensations. They also help you make facial expressions, move and blink your eyes, and move your tongue.

Developmental coordination disorder	DCD is another diagnostic name given to the symptoms of apraxia. Children with DCD struggle to master simple motor activities and are unable to perform many self-care or age-appropriate motor tasks. Though they usually have normal or above average intellectual ability, their motor coordination challenges may impact their academic progress, social interactions and emotional development. Some children may experience difficulties in a multitude of areas while others may have problems with only specific things.
Dysregulation	The state in which a person is unable to control or "regulate" their own emotional or physical response to stimuli around them. It may also be described as a dramatic fluctuation in mood or emotions resulting in anger outbursts, injurious actions towards oneself or others, or other damaging behaviors.
Elizabeth Torres	Dr. Elizabeth Torres is a highly regarded and well-published researcher on the faculty of Rutgers University. The author of several studies, many of which are compiled in her book *Autism: The Movement Sensing Perspective*, she and colleagues aim to create an alternative unifying data-driven framework grounded in physiological factors to identify and treat autism and its sensory-movement-based components. Rather than the prevailing social-emotional deficit model of diagnosis, Dr. Torres is showing how the identification of the source of these sensory-motor deficits can lead to the design of therapies that improve motor learning and performance in activities of everyday life. Her ultimate goal is to contribute to the science that improves communication as well as social opportunities in autistic children.

Executive attention	Executive attention is the ability to hold a thought (or answer) in your mind while you execute a motor task. It involves choosing what you will pay attention to and what you will ignore. In layman's terms, this is often called concentration or attentional control. In the case of a speller with sensory-motor differences, they often experience internal and external stimuli differently than a neurotypical individual and, as a result, may experience more distractions while attempting to start or finish a motor plan.
	Though we do not coach a person's intellect in Spellers Method, we sometimes coach students to "hold on to" their idea or the phrase they intend to spell as they start the sequence of spelling. This is only meant to bring focus to their executive attention skills, as it relates to motor planning, and to support them in strengthening this important ability.
Fight or flight	Fight or flight refers to reactionary states of arousal that our primitive ancestors used to survive threatening situations. Although we rarely find ourselves being chased by tigers in the twenty-first century, these automatic responses to stressful situations have been passed down to us through evolution. They are instinctive, survival-based modes that trigger the sympathetic nervous system to prepare the body to either fight or escape any threatening situation at hand.
Fine motor	Fine motor refers to motor movements that involve small muscles in the body. This includes activities like writing, cutting with scissors, holding a pencil, buttoning or zipping clothes, doing a puzzle, and moving the eyes to scan a letterboard.

Fixation	Fixation is the capacity of the eyes to maintain a steady and concentrated gaze on a specific target without moving off. This is an ocular motor task that is achieved through coordinating and controlling the different muscles and nerves that are necessary for eye movement. In regards to spelling, fixation is important for keeping the eyes locked in on each letter so the speller can maintain eye gaze and poke accurately, but fixation also plays a role in activities like reading, tracking moving objects, and sustaining visual attention.
Fluency	Fluency is the stage of letterboard communication that involves mastery of three different components: the level of communication achieved (from answering known questions to open questions), the number of CPs the speller is open with (expanded from spelling solely with the practitioner, to adding a parent as a CP, to working with two or more CPs), and the setting that the student is able to spell in (from being isolated in a room, to a room with distractions, to spelling outside).
Fluent	A "fluent" speller refers to a student who is able to spell openly with two or more CPs (communication regulation partners) in any setting.
Frontal lobe	The frontal lobe is the area of the brain where the motor cortex lies. It is important for voluntary movement, expressive language and for managing higher level executive functions.
Gestural prompt	Gestural prompts are slight hand gestures made with the left hand in the direction of the next letter that is being spelled. Gestural prompts can only be applied during spell worlds and known questions because that is when there is only one answer. It is imperative to *not* use gestural prompts during open-ended answers. Doing so is considered influencing the speller.
Gross motor	Gross motor refers to motor movements that involve large muscle groups of the body. This includes activities like walking, kicking, jumping, climbing, swinging a bat, and poking on a letterboard.

IEP	IEP is an acronym for "Individualized Education Program." This is a legal document used in the United States school system for students with disabilities who require accommodations due to a qualifying diagnosis. Developed by a comprehensive team including the parents, teacher, speech therapist, school psychologist, etc., this document lays out the student's present levels of academic performance, goals, and all accommodations and services needed.
Initiation prompt	Initiation prompts are a combination of words and/or gestures used to get the speller's movement started. Lowering the letterboard down in front of the speller's dominant spelling hand is an initiation prompt in itself, but the speller also needs a strong verbal prompt paired with that motion. The CP starts by placing the board down in front of the speller while giving a strong verbal cue such as "go get it" or "first letter is . . ." The combination of placing the board down paired with the verbal prompt aids in kick-starting the speller's movement.
Intentional movement (or intentional motor)	Intentional motor is one of the four types of motor movements (which also include automatic, impulsive, and reflexive movement). Intentional motor movement uses the cortical region of the brain (the "thinking" region), in order to act purposefully. As an intentional movement is practiced over and over again, it becomes myelinated in the brain and eventually becomes an automatic motor movement. An example of this is learning to drive a car: In the beginning, a new driver is hyperaware of all of the different components of driving (seat belt, mirror positioning, speed, use of the blinker, driving within the lines, paying attention to street signs, pedestrians, other cars, etc.). These motor movements are done purposefully, with much thinking and effort involved. With time and practice, these motor movements become automatic (faster, with less thinking and effort needed).

	Spelled communication targets the use of intentional motor skills to purposefully scan a letterboard and poke the desired letters correctly, with the idea that consistent practice will lead to this form of communication becoming less effortful and more automatic.
Interoception	One of the lesser known senses, interoception, is the process of how the brain takes in, interprets, and then integrates and assigns meaning to internal signals from the body, consciously or subconsciously. Interoception signals include: temperature regulation, pain perception, gastrointestinal (GI) sensations, emotions, or the ability to feel thirst or hunger. Individuals with autism and apraxia may have challenges perceiving one or more of these internal signals making it difficult to regulate on their own.
Least dangerous assumption	The least dangerous assumption is a concept coined by respected researcher Anne Donnellan that states that "in the absence of conclusive data educational decisions ought to be based on assumptions which, if incorrect, will have the least dangerous effect on the likelihood that students will be able to function independently as adults." The least dangerous assumption is to presume (competence) that all students want to learn and can learn when taught appropriately. https://doi.org/10.1177/019874298400900201
Minimal speaker	A minimal speaker is anyone who identifies as such and has limited speech. While the amount of verbal output may vary from person to person (one word versus fifty words, for example), it is not enough speech to fully communicate their thoughts, feelings, and ideas to the world. For these individuals, speech cannot be relied upon to robustly communicate.
Motor	Often used synonymously in the world of spelling to mean muscle movement, or the execution of a series of muscle movements. For example, "coaching the motor" means to verbally coach a student to move their muscles through a series of steps.

Motor cortex	The motor cortex is the region of the brain responsible for the planning, control, and execution of voluntary motor movements (praxis). It is divided into two parts, the primary motor cortex and the non-primary motor cortex.
Motor loops	A "motor loop" is a term we use to describe a repetitive movement that may or may not be intentional. It is an automatic movement that has been practiced over and over which has resulted in a well myelinated neural pathway between the brain and the moving body part(s).
Motor skill	Motor skills are the abilities that allow us to carry out various movements and activities in our daily lives with intention and purpose. Motor skills rely on the capacity to perceive and be aware of the actions that are being performed by our muscles during the movement process.
Multi-modal communicator	A multi-modal communicator refers to someone who communicates through a variety of methods; this includes but is not limited to: spelling as communication, gestures, speech, AAC devices, and sign language.
Myelinated	Myelin is an insulating layer, or sheath that forms around nerves, including those in the brain and spinal cord. It is made up of protein and fatty substances. When neural pathways are *myelinated,* it means all the synaptic connections are covered in a myelin sheath allowing the electrical impulses to transmit quickly and efficiently along the nerve cells. In the case of neural pathways for movement, this also results in more efficient motor output.
Neuroception	Per Dr. Stephen Porges, neuroception is the process by which our reptilian or primitive brain receives incoming sensory information from our environment. This information tells us whether the situation at hand is safe or not. Based upon this information, our body responds in a number of different ways.

Neuroplasticity	Neuroplasticity is the ability of the brain to form and reorganize its structure, function, and synaptic connections, especially in response to learning, or experience, or following injury. Essentially, it's the power of the human brain to adapt and develop new neural pathways resulting in restored or even new functionality. https://www.ncbi.nlm.nih.gov/books /NBK557811/
Neuroreceptors	Neuroreceptors are tiny protein structures that receive information from neurotransmitters, or chemical messengers, throughout the body. They facilitate communication between different parts of the body and the brain. When they receive information from a neurotransmitter, they signal other parts of the body or nervous system into action.
Nonspeaker	For the purposes of this book, a nonspeaker is anyone who identifies as such, and has either no speech, minimal speech, or unreliable speech. They cannot rely on their verbal output to fully communicate their thoughts, feelings, and ideas to the world.
Ocular motor	Ocular motor refers to the movement of the eyes. This is a form of fine motor movement, as it involves the tiny and highly complicated muscles needed to move the eyes.
Open	An "open" speller refers to a student who is able to express their own original thoughts, ideas, and feelings through spelling on a 26 letterboard (either a laminate, stencil, or keyboard). Becoming open requires working along the cognitive and motor continuums until the student is able to cleanly spell answering open questions on a full letterboard containing the entire alphabet. "Open" questions in a spelling lesson are those that ask a speller to share their own thoughts and feelings. The answer is unknown to the CP, and therefore the CP cannot use any gestural or directional prompts that will influence the speller's answer.

OT	OT is an acronym for occupational therapist. This is a highly trained professional who works to support an individual's ability to do the things they want and need to do in life. This can include activities of daily living such as eating, showering, going to the bathroom, getting dressed, job-related skills, sports, hobbies, and so much more.
PECS™	PECS is an acronym for Picture Exchange Communication System. This is an AAC system for individuals who cannot rely on speech to communicate and is frequently taught to young children with nonspeaking autism. The communicator selects a picture or symbol card from a field of options to convey a message and exchanges that picture card with their intended communication partner.
Polyvagal theory	Polyvagal theory, developed by Stephen W. Porges, was first introduced in 1994. It takes its name from the vagus nerve, which is the primary component of the parasympathetic nervous system. The traditional view of the autonomic nervous system presents a two-part system: the sympathetic nervous system, which triggers a "fight or flight" response, and the parasympathetic nervous system, which supports health, growth, and restoration, also known as the "rest and digest" state. Polyvagal theory identifies a third type of nervous system response—the social engagement system, a hybrid state of activation and calming that plays a role in our ability to socially engage (or not).

Praxis	Praxis is the complex process by which we are able to perform voluntary ("purposeful") motor movements in order to smoothly and successfully interact with our environment. This process begins with the ideation of a motor action (e.g., "I want to take a drink of my coffee"), then planning, sequencing, and organizing the motor movements needed to execute that action (e.g., the eyes move to the coffee mug, the arm reaches out, the fingers open up, the fingers close around the mug, the arm contracts towards the body and lifts the mug to the mouth, etc.), the actual execution of this motor plan, and adaptation of the motor plan as needed.
Presuming competence	Presuming competence is the belief that the person(s) you are working with has the ability to think, learn, and understand even if they cannot demonstrate their knowledge. The presumption of competence is the foundation of spelling and working with individuals with apraxia.
Primary motor cortex	The motor cortex is divided into two parts, the primary motor cortex and the nonprimary motor cortex. The primary motor cortex is critical for initiating motor movements. The nonprimary motor cortex, which further divides into other areas such as the premotor and supplementary cortex, is involved with planning, initiating, and selecting the correct movement.
Proprioception	Proprioception is the body's ability to know where it is in space. When your proprioceptive system is not working effectively, you may seek out input and pressure to activate the receptors in your muscles to reorient your body.
Proprioceptors	We have proprioceptors, or specialized sensory receptors in our bodies, that send information to the brain so we know how to respond in movement or positioning of the body. For example, proprioceptors inform our muscles on how much force to use when we are holding something or how to position our body when rock climbing.

RAS (reticular activating system)	The reticular activating system is a network of neurons that can be found in the brain stem. One of its primary roles is to help filter the bombardment of sensory stimuli that our brains are exposed to minute by minute and let through to our cortical brain only that which warrants our attention. The RAS helps to mediate behavior, stimulate our wake-sleep transitions, and is integral to our attention and consciousness.
Regulation	In the simplest terms, regulation means managing yourself. It's having the ability to recognize your internal needs, make good decisions in the moment, and respond to your emotions in adaptive ways. When regulated, a person feels a sense of balance. This state can be described as feeling calm, alert, ready and available for engaging with others.
Reinforcer	A reinforcer is anything that your speller enjoys (praise, hugs, candy, preferred toys, etc.) that when provided following the occurrence of a behavior increases the probability that the behavior will increase or happen again.
RPM	Soma®RPM (Soma-Rapid Prompting Method) also known as RPM, is a teaching method founded by Soma Mukhopadhyay. It is an academic program leading towards communication, the expression of reasoning and understanding, more reliable motor skills, and greater sensory tolerance. These goals are achieved through spelled communication. For more information visit https://www.halo-soma.org/.
S2C	Spelling to Communicate—S2C Spelling to Communicate, founded by Elizabeth Vosseller, is a form of spelled communication. It teaches students to point to letters to spell as an alternative means of communication (AAC). As motor skills improve through practice, students progress from pointing to letters on letterboards to typing on a keyboard. Accordingly, communication moves from concrete to abstract as motor skills progress. For more information visit www.I-ASC.org.

Saccadic eye movements	Saccadic eye movements are purposeful, quick, and small eye movements from one stationary object to another.
SCERTS	The SCERTS® Model is a research-based educational approach and multidisciplinary framework that directly addresses the core challenges faced by children and persons with ASD and related disabilities, and their families. SCERTS® focuses on building competence in social communication, emotional regulation and transactional support as the highest priorities that must be addressed in any program, and is applicable for individuals with a wide range of abilities and ages across home, school and community settings. For more information visit https://scerts.com/.
Sensory foam letterboards	Sensory foam boards are a type of letterboard with craft alphabet letters glued onto a foam board background. These can be made in a set of three boards (A-I, J-R, S-Z) as well as the full alphabet board with all twenty-six letters on one. They provide a stronger visual contrast between the letter and the background versus the stencil letters, and can be especially useful for younger spellers or students who cannot grasp a pencil or stylus.
Sensory integration disorder (SID)	Sensory integration disorder (SID) or sensory processing disorder (SPD) are neurological disorders that result from the brain's inability to integrate certain information received from the body's sensory systems.
Sensory integration theory	Sensory integration theory was developed by A. Jean Ayres based on her knowledge of neuroscience and occupational therapy. In treatment, it involves the client working with an OT and participating in individualized activities that aim to improve deficits within the individual's sensory integration functioning.

SLP	SLP is an acronym for speech-language pathologist. Commonly referred to as a "speech therapist," this is a professional with a master's degree in communication disorders, specializing in the assessment, prevention, and treatment of communication and swallowing disorders.
Smooth pursuits	Smooth pursuits are tracking eye movements where the eyes maintain fixation on a moving object.
Supplementary motor cortex	The SMC is the part of the motor cortex involved in planning and learning new motor sequences.
Synaptic connections	Synaptic connections, or synapses, are the places where neurons connect and communicate with each other. Each neuron has anywhere between a few to hundreds of thousands of synaptic connections, and these connections can be with itself, neighboring neurons, or neurons in other regions of the brain.
Top-down regulation	Top-down regulation involves helping a student feel calm and available to engage by employing strategies that are more cognitive-based. These strategies require the speller to think and process what they are hearing. Mindfulness practices, guided visualizations, reading high cognitive lessons, or playing educational podcasts in the background are all top-down regulation strategies.
Unreliable speaker	An unreliable speaker is someone who has speech, but may repeatedly use certain words and phrases without intending to. This can include "scripting"—repeating lines heard from a show, movie, etc., "echolalia"— repeating back words heard from another person, and "verbal loops"—often repeating certain words or phrases, not usually with purpose; getting stuck repeating the same thing. The individual's speech cannot always be relied upon for them to communicate purposefully what they're thinking.

Vagus nerve	The vagus nerve is the longest of the twelve cranial nerves in the body. It runs from the brain stem (the primitive brain) to the large intestine and is responsible for all sorts of automatic activities like heart rate, breathing, digestion, and reflexive actions such as sneezing, swallowing, and vomiting. It plays a critical role in activating the parasympathetic nervous system.
Vestibular system	The vestibular system gives the body its sense of balance. It works in conjunction with receptors in the inner ear as well as the visual system to keep the body upright.
Wernicke's area	A region of the brain that is primarily responsible for comprehension. Located in the cerebral cortex, Wernicke's area is connected to Broca's area via neural pathways and contains the neurons necessary for comprehending and understanding speech and written language.

Bibliography

Coulter, R. A. et al. "Near-point Findings in Children with Autism Spectrum Disorder and in Typical Peers." *Optometry and Vision Science* 98, no. 4 (2021), 384-393. https://doi.org/10.1097/OPX.0000000000001679

Donnellan, A. M. (1984). The Criterion of the Least Dangerous Assumption. Behavioral Disorders, 9(2), 141–150. https://doi.org/10.1177/019874298400900201

Kaplan, M., B. Rimland, and S. M. Edelson. "Strabismus in Autism Spectrum Disorder." *Focus on Autism and Other Developmental Disabilities* 14, no. 2 (1999), 101-105. https://doi.org/10.1177/108835769901400205

Kemner, C. et al. "Are Abnormal Event-Related Potentials Specific to Children with ADHD? A Comparison with Two Clinical Groups. *Perceptual and Motor Skills* 87, no. 3 (1998), 1083-1090. https://doi.org/10.2466/pms.1998.87.3.1083

Leekam SR, Nieto C, Libby SJ, Wing L, Gould J. Describing the sensory abnormalities of children and adults with autism. *J Autism Dev Disord.* 2007 May;37(5):894-910. doi: 10.1007/s10803-006-0218-7. PMID: 17016677.

Scharre, Janice Emigh and Margaret Procyk Creedon. "Assessment of Visual Function in Autistic Children." *Optometry and Vision Science*, 69, no. 6 (1992), 433-439. https://doi.org/10.1097/00006324-199206000-00004

Simmons, David R. et al. "Vision in Autism Spectrum Disorders." *Vision Research* 49, no. 22 (2009), 2705-2739. https://doi.org/10.1016/j.visres.2009.08.005

Takarae, Yukari et al. "Pursuit Eye Movement Deficits in Autism." *Brain: A Journal of Neurology* 127, no. 12 (2004), 2584-2594. https://doi.org/10.1093/brain/awh307

Torres Elizabeth, Brincker Maria, Isenhower Robert, Yanovich Polina, Stigler
Kimberly, Nurnberger John I, Metaxas Dimitri, Jose Jorge. Autism: the
micro-movement perspective. *Frontiers in Integrative Neuroscience,* 7 (2013).
https://www.frontiersin.org/articles/10.3389/fnint.2013.00032 DOI=10.3389
/fnint.2013.00032

Torres, E. & Whyatt, C. (2020). Autism: The movement Sensing Perspective.
Frontiers in Neuroscience.

Appendix A

BOOKS WRITTEN BY SPELLERS AND TYPERS

TITLE	AUTHOR	LINK
Anatomy of Autism: A Pocket Guide for Educators, Parents, and Students	Diego Pena	https://www.amazon.com/Anatomy -Autism-Educators-Parents -Students/dp/1544038089/ref=pd _bxgy_14_img_3/145-5510921 -1441949?_encoding=UTF8&pd _rd_i=1544038089&pd_rd_r =1f899a5d-7bd2-4186-bc1a -10ec8b0dc4d2&pd_rd_w=cn4Le &pd_rd_wg=XEXJ2&pf_rd_p =09627863-9889-4290-b90a -5e9f86682449&pf_rd_r =NCTMT21S77MYT10STZPM &psc=1&refRID =NCTMT21S77MYT10STZPM
AUTISTIC & AWESOME: A Journal from the Inside	Alfonso Julian Camacho	https://www.amazon.com /AUTISTIC-AWESOME-Alfonso -Juli%C3%A1n-Camacho-ebook /dp/B07QYLQH8V/ref=sr_1_1 ?dchild=1&keywords=camacho +autism&qid=1607705974&sr =8-1&pldnSite=1

Continued

TITLE	AUTHOR	LINK
Carly's Voice: Breaking Through Autism	Arthur Fleischmann	https://www.amazon.com/Carlys-Voice-Breaking-Through-Autism-ebook/dp/B005FLOEGA/ref=pd_sim_351_2/145-5510921-1441949?_encoding=UTF8&pd_rd_i=B005FLOEGA&pd_rd_r=1ab4aece-d9c0-4455-b1c4-9305eef08cd8&pd_rd_w=DrOGK&pd_rd_wg=WOEjt&pf_rd_p=5abf8658-0b5f-405c-b880-a6d1b558d4ea&pf_rd_r=6FT6FDW30JVHXZDH4YVA&psc=1&refRID=6FT6FDW30JVHXZDH4YVA
Communication Alternatives in Autism: Perspectives on Typing and Spelling Approaches for the Nonspeaking	Edlyn Vallejo Pena	https://www.amazon.com/Communication-Alternatives-Autism-Perspectives-Nonspeaking/dp/147667891X/ref=pd_bxgy_14_img_2/145-5510921-1441949?_encoding=UTF8&pd_rd_i=147667891X&pd_rd_r=aa7b70be-ff66-4285-be0e-fed440090610&pd_rd_w=iMiJ8&pd_rd_wg=phtFG&pf_rd_p=09627863-9889-4290-b90a-5e9f86682449&pf_rd_r=R5A145BM4P5VRGF27ZYJ&psc=1&refRID=R5A145BM4P5VRGF27ZYJ
Danson: The Extraordinary Discovery of an Autistic Child's Innermost Thoughts and Feelings	Michele Pierce Burns and Danson Mandela Wambua	https://www.amazon.com/Danson-Extraordinary-Discovery-Autistic-Innermost/dp/0980028841/ref=sr_1_1?dchild=1&keywords=danson%20mandela%20wambua&qid=1617583917&s=books&sr=1-1&fbclid=IwAR0aSM67h8yqCkTpGqLIFp4fUVZWG-nA5JHTc_mczV0weJsG6sA0rp3bgKg

Continued

TITLE	AUTHOR	LINK
DETECTIVE NICK AND THE CASE OF THE MISSING BELLY BUTTONS: Investigating the Weird and Unusual	Nicholas A. Milivojevich	https://www.amazon.com/ DETECTIVE-NICK-MISSING -BELLY-BUTTONS/dp/B08RCG3S76 /ref=sr_1_3?dchild=1&keywords =Detective+Nick&qid =1616699933&sr=8-3
Eating Broccoli on the Moon	Dustin Duby-Koffman	https://www.unrestrictedinterest .com/reading/p/eating-broccoli-on -the-moon-by-dustin-duby-koffman
Fall Down 7 Times Get Up 8: A Young Man's Voice from the Silence of Autism	Naoki Higashida	https://www.amazon.com/Fall-Down -Times-Get-Up/dp/0812987195/ref=pd _sbs_14_2/145-5510921-1441949? _encoding=UTF8&pd_rd _i=0812987195&pd_rd_r=7277253b -c145-4fe5-bc70-8735db0b97a3&pd _rd_w=IQWk1&pd_rd_wg =fZKUo&pf_rd_p=52b7592c-2dc9 -4ac6-84d4-4bda6360045e&pf_rd_r =0DWDJRP3JWMNZSVATSS8 &psc=1&refRID =0DWDJRP3JWMNZSVATSS8
Handbook of Us: Understanding and Accepting People with Autism	Matteo Musso	https://www.amazon.com /Handbook-Us-Understanding -Accepting-People/dp/0998863629 /ref=tmm_pap_swatch_0? _encoding=UTF8&qid=&sr=
How Can I Talk If My Lips Don't Move?: Inside My Autistic Mind	Tito Rajarshi Mukhopadhyay	https://www.amazon.com/How -Talk-Lips-Dont-Move-ebook/dp /B00CKXAAKK/ref=sr_1_1?qid =1573766581&refinements=p_27 %3ATito+Rajarshi+Mukhopadhyay &s=books&sr=1-1&text=Tito +Rajarshi+Mukhopadhyay

Continued

TITLE	AUTHOR	LINK
I Am in Here: The Journey of a Child with Autism Who Cannot Speak but Finds Her Voice	Elizabeth M. Bonker and Virginia G. Breen	https://www.amazon.com/Am-Here-Journey-Autism-Cannot-ebook/dp/B005LOPOCY/ref=sr_1_1?keywords=elizabeth+bonker&qid=1573766710&s=books&sr=1-1
I Have Been Buried Under Years of Dust: A Memoir of Autism and Hope	Valeri Gilpeer and Emily Grodin	https://www.amazon.com/Have-Been-Buried-Under-Years-ebook/dp/B08CRD7CWY/ref=sr_1_1?crid=1KPELHVV1I4L0&dchild=1&keywords=i+have+been+buried+under+years+of+dust&qid=1616606045&sprefix=i+have+been+bur%2Caps%2C159&sr=8-1&pldnSite=1
I Never Get Lost in the Woods	Aaron Jepson	https://www.amazon.com/I-Never-Get-Lost-Woods/dp/1960583018/ref=sr_1_1?crid=16UACQ2GGMJKD&keywords=jepson+autism&qid=1686542899&s=books&sprefix=jepson+autism%2Cstripbooks%2C139&sr=1-1
Ido in Autismland: Climbing Out of Autism's Silent Prison	Ido Kedar	https://www.amazon.com/Ido-Autismland-Climbing-Autisms-Silent/dp/0988324709/ref=pd_sbs_14_2/145-5510921-1441949?_encoding=UTF8&pd_rd_i=0988324709&pd_rd_r=35d5ea38-c509-48bd-a741-beca36facab8&pd_rd_w=f3flg&pd_rd_wg=arSUU&pf_rd_p=52b7592c-2dc9-4ac6-84d4-4bda6360045e&pf_rd_r=NZF75SNFA8WB15HPV7XF&psc=1&refRID=NZF75SNFA8WB15HPV7XF

Continued

TITLE	AUTHOR	LINK
In Two Worlds	Ido Kedar	https://www.amazon.com/Two-Worlds-Ido-Kedar/dp/1732291500/ref=pd_bxgy_14_img_2/145-5510921-1441949?_encoding=UTF8&pd_rd_i=1732291500&pd_rd_r=0e043cf9-0bcf-4789-aaa7-2f08aa657a51&pd_rd_w=Hs7hJ&pd_rd_wg=q4Wfm&pf_rd_p=09627863-9889-4290-b90a-5e9f86682449&pf_rd_r=0FNATA2E59WQEEPQVZFV&psc=1&refRID=0FNATA2E59WQEEPQVZFV
Leaders Around Me: Autobiographies of Autistics Who Type, Point, and Spell to Communicate	Edlyn Vallejo Pena	https://www.amazon.com/Leaders-Around-Autobiographies-Autistics-Communicate/dp/1791505953/ref=sr_1_fkmr0_1?keywords=leaders+all+around+me&qid=1573766155&sr=8-1-fkmr0
Plankton Dreams: What I Learned in Special Ed	Tito Rajarshi Mukhopadhyay	https://www.amazon.com/Plankton-Dreams-What-Learned-Special/dp/1785420070/ref=sr_1_1?crid=28ZGOU7DEVVG9&keywords=tito+mukhopadhyay&qid=1573766528&s=books&sprefix=tito+m%2Cstripbooks%2C148&sr=1-1
Real	Carol Cujec and Peyton Goddard	https://www.amazon.com/Real-Carol-Cujec/dp/162972789X/ref=sr_1_1?crid=I9E4SOPUSWVA&dchild=1&keywords=peyton+goddard&qid=1616606333&sprefix=peyton+go%2Caps%2C159&sr=8-1&pldnSite=1

Continued

TITLE	AUTHOR	LINK
See It Feelingly: Classic Novels, Autistic Readers, and the Schooling of a No-Good English Professor (Thought in the Act)	Ralph James Savarese	https://www.amazon.com/See-Feelingly-Autistic-Schooling-Professor/dp/1478001305/ref=sr_1_1?keywords=Ralph+Savarese&qid=1573766784&sr=8-1
Spellbound: The Voices of the Silent	Judy Hope Chinitz	https://www.amazon.com/Spellbound-Voices-Judy-Hope-Chinitz/dp/B0C2S6NMQ2/ref=sr_1_1?crid=1EIYJ06I8RRM1&keywords=spellbound+book+autism&qid=1686542851&s=books&sprefix=spellbound+book+autism%2Cstripbooks%2C146&sr=1-1
Teaching Myself to See	Tito Mukhopadhyay	https://www.amazon.com/Teaching-Myself-See-Tito-Mukhopadhyay/dp/1953035329/ref=sr_1_1?crid=O8FJVTOUQR01&dchild=1&keywords=tito+mukhopadhyay&qid=1617574782&s=books&sprefix=Tito+%2Cstripbooks%2C143&sr=1-1
The Autistic Mind Finally Speaks: Letterboard Thoughts	Gregory Tino	https://www.amazon.com/Autistic-Mind-Finally-Speaks-Letterboard-ebook/dp/B08MDHD8GM/ref=sr_1_1?dchild=1&keywords=tino+autism&qid=1607705940&sr=8-1&pldnSite=1
The Elements	Tito Rajarshi Mukhopadhyay and Sarah Sohn	https://www.amazon.com/Elements-Tito-Rajarshi-Mukhopadhyay/dp/0359795250/ref=sr_1_1?keywords=Sarah+sohn&qid=1573766672&s=books&sr=1-1

Continued

TITLE	AUTHOR	LINK
The Mind Tree: A Miraculous Child Breaks the Silence of Autism	Tito Rajarshi Mukhopadhyay	https://www.amazon.com/Mind-Tree-Miraculous-Breaks-Silence-ebook/dp/B006NZBG6S/ref=pd_sim_351_3/145-5510921-1441949?_encoding=UTF8&pd_rd_i=B006NZBG6S&pd_rd_r=2b08c78f-6b41-494d-846f-923fb6a27e8b&pd_rd_w=4iFjo&pd_rd_wg=7X8qX&pf_rd_p=5abf8658-0b5f-405c-b880-a6d1b558d4ea&pf_rd_r=1F5J6HJVST2S47AH2VSY&psc=1&refRID=1F5J6HJVST2S47AH2VSY
The Reason I Jump: The Inner Voice of a Thirteen-Year-Old Boy with Autism	Naoki Higashida	https://www.amazon.com/Reason-Jump-Inner-Thirteen-Year-Old-Autism/dp/081298515X/ref=pd_sbs_14_3/145-5510921-1441949?_encoding=UTF8&pd_rd_i=081298515X&pd_rd_r=aa837ce9-3374-477a-be2d-78bf693f503d&pd_rd_w=6iPLe&pd_rd_wg=tGI9b&pf_rd_p=52b7592c-2dc9-4ac6-84d4-4bda6360045e&pf_rd_r=YK8NQ7WDHBBGBEXSB5BJ&psc=1&refRID=YK8NQ7WDHBBGBEXSB5BJ
Traveler's Tales: My Journey with Autism	Chammi Rajapatirana	https://www.amazon.ca/Travelers-Tales-My-Journey-Autism-ebook/dp/B017NZJ1AE?fbclid=IwAR1uIWUZ69I9n6E1AJwOCQwl42VCkZVtKAmP2-daXcYNw6CuKRgCSrCe-9E
Typed Words, Loud Voices	Edited by Amy Sequenza and Elizabeth J. Grace	https://autonomous-press.myshopify.com/products/typed-words-loud-voices

Continued

TITLE	AUTHOR	LINK
Underestimated	J.B. and Jamison Handley	https://www.amazon.com /Underestimated-Autism-Miracle -Childrens-Defense/dp/1510766367
Unrestricted Interests	Various authors and their publications	https://www.unrestrictedinterest .com/
Waves and Wind and We	Danny Whitty	https://www.unrestrictedinterest .com/reading/p/waves-and-wind -and-we-by-danny-whitty

About the Authors

DAWNMARIE (DM) GAIVIN'S STORY

My first son, Evan, was diagnosed with autism in June 2005 at 22 months of age. I had given birth to his little brother, Trey, just four months prior after an arduous eight-week stay in the hospital in preterm labor. During the first few weeks of that inpatient stay, Evan visited me multiple times a week with his dad. But over time, my excitement over his presence caused my labor to increase too dramatically, which made my doctor suspend his visits. It was a painful decision but done in the best interest of the new baby whose lung protein ratios were still testing as remarkably immature in utero.

Finally, the day arrived, and Tricky Trey, as we still affectionately call him, was born. A little bit early, but healthy as can be. Getting very little sleep, I self-discharged less than twenty-four hours after his birth to reunite our family. I'll never forget the relief I felt on that car ride home. I'd been dreaming of this moment for months and couldn't wait to snuggle my toddler. I rushed to Evan's bedroom to wake him from his nap, and as I gently entered the room, I began whispering his name. He stirred a little. My heart was bursting with anticipation of our reunion. I gingerly picked him up, singing one of our favorite songs, but when he opened his eyes to meet mine, he looked at me like he'd never seen me before. I'll never forget his cold, empty gaze. He didn't cry but he didn't smile or embrace me either. I brushed it off, justifying that he must still be tired. I squeezed him tightly for a moment before he pushed back and wiggled for me to put him down. He grabbed his lamb lovey and pacifier from his crib and left the room without glancing back at me. Two hours later, he was still wandering around the house aimlessly, not looking at me or for me, not responding to his name, not connected to me, anyone, or anything. The joyful anticipation that filled my heart on the car ride home was replaced with a cloud of confusion. Where had my little boy gone while I was in the hospital?

Four months and many assessments later, Evan received his diagnosis. The following year was a flurry of self-education, therapy appointments, early intervention, and DIR^R/Floortime^{TM} training. I wasn't expecting to be an "autism mom," but I seemed born for the challenge of learning about it, and I enjoyed imagining the infinite possibilities for Evan's future.

Then came June 2006. On the exact anniversary of Evan's diagnosis, Trey also received an autism spectrum label. In Trey's case, I witnessed the regression happening before my eyes, and it felt much more aggressive. Only thirty days after I had first noticed him not consistently responding to his name, he too was roaming around our home like a ghost. He lost all his speech, eye contact, social engagement, and affect. According to a study published in the *Journal of Developmental & Behavioral Pediatrics*, 21 percent of cases of autism start with this type of regression, and because both of my children experienced their diagnoses this way, it's all I know. I don't know what it's like to be a parent whose child is born and doesn't hit developmental milestones. Mine had been developing along typical timelines before their regressions. And both of my boys once had age-appropriate levels of speech. Evan had thirteen words by his first birthday and more than three hundred receptive words at fifteen months. But in June 2006, things went silent. Evan never regained his speech, and Trey was silent for several years. Although I had no reservations about being a mother to children with unique needs, it was simply uncharted territory on how to support two nonspeakers at once.

I know today there is a lot of criticism when parents share their emotional process around receiving a diagnosis for their child. I can understand why someone, especially a speaking autistic, would be deeply offended at the idea that a parent might grieve in these moments. Speaking just for myself, I can say this: I love my boys infinitely and wouldn't swap either of them for a different child for anything. Anyone who has ever spent time with us knows that without question. I love their uniqueness and how their brains work, and the diversity they bring to the planet. Today I feel incredibly blessed to be surrounded daily by neurodivergent clients and friends. But on the day of Trey's diagnosis, I *was* sad. I was sad simply because I feared I would never be enough for my two children. I was sad because I felt I could never help them as much as they each needed and deserved. Raising just one child with high support needs had taken the bulk of my attention the year before. What was I going to do now that there were two of them? Splitting my time, energy, and our family's resources would never allow me to maximize their opportunities.

Several months before Trey's diagnosis I asked my mother to move in to help ease my guilt. I felt like Trey was missing out on crucial social bonding during his first year of development because I was focusing so much on Evan. If you'd been a fly on the wall back in 2005 you'd have seen me crawling around on all fours, playfully wooing Evan to make even three seconds of sustained eye contact with me while I'd intermittently pop up to surprise Trey in his exersaucer and shout "peek-a-boo!!" to make him giggle. It was exhausting trying to juggle both of them, and now I had proof that Trey would need me just as much as Evan did. I was sad as I pondered what would happen to them if I couldn't help them reach their fullest potential.

That day, I needed to make some critical decisions about their future. Having two autistic children meant I had to split my time and resources between them both, so I figured I should prioritize my dreams. I sat in Trey's nursery for two days pondering my bottom line. What was the "must-have" impact I needed to make in their lives to set them up for future success?

As the action-oriented individual I am, I boiled it down to a short list. If I could accomplish nothing else, I wanted to make sure my children would develop relationships, become literate, find a way to communicate their wants, needs, and feelings, as well as refuse people and choices they didn't want. Lacking the vocabulary then that I have now, I essentially wanted them to have agency to self-determine their adult lives and have relationships of their choosing someday. That meant doing a lot of social-emotional-based therapy and turning over every rock until they both could communicate effectively.

Our AAC (augmentative and alternative communication) journey began at home with PECS, SCERTS, a single switch called the "Big Mac" to teach Evan the power of words and an amazing special ed preschool teacher named Wendy Burkhardt. Even though the district AT specialist told us Evan wasn't capable, Wendy believed in him and presumed competence. When we purchased and delivered the first HP touchscreen computer to her classroom, she practiced with Evan several times a week so he would learn to visually scan and select icons with an isolated finger to communicate his choices. Without realizing it, she was coaching his motor, so he could eventually start showing us what he truly understood. This presumption of competence—a willingness and ability to learn—is a hallmark principle of spelling for communication. But more on that later.

From there, he had an independent assistive technology (AT) assessment which showed he *would* benefit from an SGD (speech-generating device), and we started our journey using the Vantage-Lite, made by PRC. I was intuitively drawn to this device because of the concept behind LAMP (Language Acquisition through Motor Planning), their software that takes into careful consideration the dyspraxic nonspeaker's experience. The placement of the icons is not dependent on the whim or preference of the person programming it. Instead, it is preprogrammed and the buttons are always in the same place. Once Evan learned the motor plan required to sequence a phrase or sentence, he could execute it more and more consistently on his own.

Flash forward to 2012. Evan was attending a nonpublic special education program paid for by our school district and was using his SGD to meet many of his IEP (Individualized Education Program) goals. Evan could use it to speak phrases but generally limited his conversation to requesting needs and wants. Though practical, I had aspirations for more robust communication. So I started working feverishly at home to teach him how to spell. I mistakenly thought this was a prerequisite to trying RPM, Rapid Prompting Method, a trademarked methodology that Soma Mukhopadhyay developed. Per her website, RPM is an academic program for autistic students that often leads to communication. In my copious research this felt like the last stone to turn over in my quest for Evan to be able to express himself robustly. After all, I believed if he could learn to spell with all twenty-six letters in order to accomplish academics, he could also use that skill to tell us anything!

Evan today muses about that time in our life. In the short chapter he wrote in Jamie and J. B. Handley's book *Underestimated*, he talks about how relieved he was when I finally "realized [he] didn't need to prove [he] could spell" before I'd buckle down to teach him this form of alternative communication. Evan says he knew how to spell long before that time. In fact, he says he could spell by age two, but he could not arrange the one-inch plastic letter tiles onto the pictures I had carefully selected and laminated. Not only were the materials flat on the table, which later I would learn was very difficult for Evan's eyes to scan, but he had to execute precise fine motor skills to move the tiles properly. He didn't lack cognition. He needed to gain the motor planning ability to show me that he could already spell and read.

Despite him failing my makeshift "home spelling training," I ended up hosting a Level 2 RPM Practitioner for a weekend in 2015. I signed both Evan and Trey up for sessions with this well-respected teacher. I watched this expert clinician interact with my restless duo and get them to successfully poke letters in stencils to spell out words. Because I was the host for this outreach, I also sat in on all the other students' sessions and furiously dissected what I was observing in my mind. I saw that the materials used in each lesson were the same, but the application was unique based on each student's profile. On the one hand, that made perfect sense to me, because if you've met one person with autism, you've met only one person with autism. But on the other hand, this individualized approach made it challenging to know how to replicate the method with my two sons. Nonetheless, I was encouraged enough to move forward. I bought all of Soma's books, voraciously read them, and started spelling for at least ten minutes daily with Evan. I also began reading age-appropriate literature to them every night. After all, if writing was going to be their primary method of communication, they needed to understand how words go together to make sentences, and how sentences go together to make paragraphs. They also needed a robust vocabulary beyond the core words we all use to generically communicate most basic information.

The first two weeks after the outreach, I tried spelling with both boys. My biggest obstacle was that I had recently become a single mom and found the lesson prep and practice time required made life a little unmanageable. I accepted that doing my best as a mother would mean trying to ensure fair, but not necessarily equal, resource allocation to my children. So I decided to start just with Evan. I chose E because he never regained speech after his initial regression whereas Trey had regained some and was minimally verbal. Tricky Trey would have to wait just a bit longer for his time on the boards.

Six months later, this same practitioner returned to San Diego for another outreach I hosted. Once again, I sat in on all the sessions to observe and soak in what I could. Evan spelled his first "open" thoughts that week. Short and sweet but mind-blowing nonetheless. When discussing a poem that stated, "the sunlight warmed the boy's skin like God's love," the teacher asked Evan, "what's another word for God's love?" I looked at my occupational therapy (OT) colleague Vicky Golden sitting beside me, and we both shrugged. If neither of us could think of a synonym, how would he? Evan then spelled out the word *benevolent*. My jaw dropped. He was only twelve years old. What twelve-year-old uses that word? Incidentally, I have since adopted this term as my name for God: the Benevolent Universe. But back to that day, Evan also randomly commented to the teacher, "I think my mom is smart." That was the first thing he had ever said to me. The kind teacher agreed with him.

Another six months later, through my professional DIR/Floortime™ connections, I was invited to a small workshop at Cal Lutheran University being offered by Elizabeth Vosseller, the founder of S2C. In this life-changing three-day intensive, I learned the science behind apraxia, the foundations of spelling to communicate, and even had practice sessions with nonspeakers who were already fluent spellers. The benevolent universe graciously paired me that day with speller and Cal Lutheran graduate, Samuel Capozzi. To say I was fangirling and nervous is an understatement. He and his beautiful family were such inspirations to me, and I looked to them for many years (and still do) for guidance both as a mom and a communication partner for my son.

At that point, I had never spelled with anyone except my boys. Sam was so patient and encouraging that I was inspired to become a practitioner. Luckily, Elizabeth was starting a training program through her private practice later that same year. By the fall of 2016, Evan was spelling openly with me, largely thanks to the standardization I learned at EV's workshop, which built upon the promising motor start I had practicing RPM for a year. And in March 2017, I began my training as an S2C practitioner.

Since then, I've voraciously read white papers, research articles, books, and blogs of nonspeakers, trying to understand all the subtleties that go into nonspeaking autistics' experiences. I've become an assistive technology specialist and taken multiple graduate-level courses in both autism curriculum design as well as marriage and family therapy. But it is truly from the spelled words of my nonspeaking clients that I have learned the most. Largely in part to the incredible book *Underestimated* by Jamie and J. B. Handley, my tiny practice has grown from one practitioner with eight (very special) clients to multiple practitioners and more than five hundred clients in just a few years. In 2021, I joined forces with Dana Johnson, PhD, OTR/L who was running an equally large clinical practice in Florida and we began a company called Empowered2 which was dedicated to supporting parents and caregivers of nonspeakers as key stakeholders in their loved one's communication journey. We created the first online Communication Partner (CP) training program to help meet the needs of new spellers who couldn't find local practitioners and we ran several week-long immersion programs with the same goal in mind. Our CP courses now run continuously in eight-week cohorts and are supporting spellers all over the world to get on the boards and begin their life-changing journey. In 2022 we rebranded all of our entities together under one name and Spellers was born.

By running two of the largest spelling centers in the country, we have seen students with a wide variety of sensory-motor profiles come through our doors. Since we first met ten years ago, Dana and I have been researching various theories around dyspraxia, ocular motor differences, and intentional motor programs to better support non-speakers. The results we have seen with our spelling clients have been truly inspirational. We have applied what we learned from our decades of professional experience to our current clinical judgments, making communication accessible to each student. At times, this requires some individualization, which I initially observed in RPM. This also requires a systematic approach to gradually increasing the motor and cognitive demands of communication, which we both observed in S2C. But it is through our training, backgrounds, research, and experience with our own clients we have trialed and discovered a precise order of operations to affect our typers' future autonomy.

Though we admit it's an assumption, we believe a primary goal of every human is to achieve a life of self-determination. If that's true, then all spellers must learn the skills needed—both on and off the boards—to control their bodies, communicate (hopefully without a communication partner someday), and be free to express their wishes and dreams. This is why the Spellers Method was born. The multidisciplinary approach to spelled communication and intentional movement is the foundation for a life of autonomy for nonspeakers.

DANA JOHNSON'S STORY

For as long as I can remember I have wanted to help people. Specifically working with children was something that I felt drawn to doing. When I was young, I envisioned myself later on in life with a family and thought that working with children would be good practice. I volunteered in every way I could—church programs, after school programs, sports leagues, and even summer camps. One year I had the fortunate opportunity to be the summer director of the special needs camp at a sports resort in Ontario, Canada. It changed my life. There I met an amazing boy named Owen. He had been there in previous years but this was the first year I was heading up the camp so it was our first year together. He wore a tie-dyed T-shirt and gym shorts every day. I learned that this was so he could easily be identified because as I was told he was autistic and runs away—fast!

Owen was the first individual that I met with nonspeaking autism and he and I hung out along with his 1:1 counselor that summer. I learned so much from Owen over those weeks. He was smart, even though most people didn't believe he was able to understand (at that time I didn't think he fully understood either), he was creative (art, specifically painting, was his gift), and he had a way of truly enjoying the nature around him. I took a few minutes to observe him one day and he seemed to soak in every single detail of the woods around him. He didn't care about the world around him. He was literally "stopping to smell the roses" or in his case "stopping to pick up dead leaves because of the certain shape and angle" and was enjoying every single minute of it! To this day when I think about that, I wish I stopped more often to take in and appreciate what is around me like he did.

Fast forward a couple of years later and I was fully engulfed in courses to complete my Master's in Occupational Therapy. I continued to think about Owen and all that he taught me that summer, but I had also met other autistic people who I connected with along the way. I read and studied everything I could about autism and the research that surrounded this diagnosis that at the time affected 1 in 150 children. I organized my internships, papers, and classes so that I could learn as much as possible about why this diagnosis was affecting so many. I would stay up late at night reviewing research papers on autism and how it affects children's ability to interact socially, maintain eye contact, and learn (little did I know how much that would change in the years ahead!). I specifically dove into the research surrounding sensory processing and how the brain of an autistic person is wired differently affecting the ability to process incoming sensory information. As a result, they can become very dysregulated. They need sensory input and specific sensory-based interventions so they can be productive, or so I read. As I continued to read, I made it my mission to build a practice devoted to not only supporting individuals with autism but also making the world a better place for them.

After graduating with my Master of Science in Occupational Therapy I took a job in the local school district because that is all I could find at the time related to pediatrics and autism. In Canada, private practice OT clinics were few and far between mainly because insurance didn't cover any OT for children outside of the school system. This is not surprising given the state of the healthcare system, but I digress. The position landed me in up to eight different schools. I had a caseload of almost fifty students between the eight schools. As you can imagine, it was clearly impossible to see them all and put the time into supporting their needs. I grew increasingly frustrated because I knew there was more that could be done to help them, but I was so limited, mainly with time. I also remember seeing the students in the "autism unit" as they call it wandering around the classroom without purpose.

My job in the schools was to provide the students with support so they could "access their curriculum." That meant if they couldn't write, attempt a handwriting program, and if that didn't work then get them a computer so they could type. That was it. Over and over again I got referrals for students with "fine motor difficulties" who couldn't take notes so I would slap a Band-Aid on the problem and hope for the best. It was not what I imagined I would be doing as my career. Yes, I was working with kids and please know, I knew these kids needed me and support, but working against a system that didn't truly support them took its toll. I began to get frustrated. This wasn't "just a job" for me, this was a passion and I soon realized it wasn't a good fit for me.

After my first year in the school system, I wanted to explore other options. I was living in Canada and it was the middle of February and it was -40 degrees Celsius. I remember asking myself *Why am I here?* I made the decision right then and there, I'm moving. I studied and wrote my US OT licensing exam and wound up in Cary, North Carolina, at a small private occupational and speech therapy clinic. Not only was it in this beautiful town and state, it was also focused on working with children with autism. I felt I had landed my dream job! Working with kids doing what I love and what I knew best.

It was there that I was introduced to a therapy called Applied Behavior Analysis or ABA. The analytical side of me thought it was great because of all the data and how progress was demonstrated. When reading so many research articles and knowing how import-ant that is, I jumped right in. As I continued to work with my clients, I questioned the methods of what I was doing more and more each day. It just didn't "feel" right. What I was trying to get my clients to do seemed *so* challenging. They would work so hard for a cookie or a few minutes with a toy. It just seemed to me like training rather than skill-building. Don't get me wrong, I made it fun and there were lots of laughs, but it seemed forced and not of their own volition. Yet this was the most researched and "the gold standard" of therapy for autistic kids so why would I question it? But I did. I needed to understand what I was doing and also feel that whatever intervention I was implementing aligned with my values. ABA did not and I knew that I had to figure out what I was going to do because I couldn't continue to practice this way.

Enter DIR/Floortime, a relationship-based way to build engagement and interaction with the child. This is what resonated with me. Letting the child lead, following what they choose while building in therapeutic intervention. I loved it! It seems so empowering for not only the child but the family. It was when I was introduced to DIR/FT that I learned the importance of the parent/caregiver role in therapy. It was the missing piece to what I knew was the best for the child and their development and progress. I continued to build my client caseload and was able to work with so many families doing what I loved to do—support the child and coach parents so they not only understood their child better but could also implement the therapeutic approaches at home. I really felt that I had my dream job. Then I met the person that would change all that—my husband. It's crazy what love does to a person but for me, it took me farther south to a state where I thought people only went to for spring break, not to live! Florida would be my new home with new beginnings. I began working in an outpatient hospital setting which quickly brought back memories of the school system. I didn't feel connected to the families; parents would just drop off their kids and take the hour to catch up on emails, and I was extremely limited in what I could do to support the child. It was all about what insurance would cover and none of it included parent/caregiver coaching and support. I lasted one year.

I opened my private practice in 2009 and have never looked back. That year I also started my PhD (I would never recommend starting a business and starting a PhD at the same time by the way!) and focused on the parent-child relationship dynamics. I am and always will be a lifelong learner and I wanted to put into practice what I had learned and experienced in the past and what I was currently learning in my PhD program. For the first time, I felt that I was doing what I had set out to do so many years before. I continued to see families and work with their children and before long I had a few families ask me to consider starting a school based on the DIR/Floortime intervention and family-based coaching that I was doing at the clinic. It would encompass academic learning and education goals but also provide therapy and family support. Sure, why not? Again, my adventurous heart dove in without knowing anything about how to start a school and or how to teach students with different learning needs.

I knew I would figure it out and I did by building my own relationships with experts in the field including Shelley Carnes, the founder and executive director of The Hirsch Academy in Atlanta, Georgia. She was not only an OT and had done this before, she also became one of my mentors and friends. She graciously welcomed me to the school over and over again to take in their model, which was based on DIR/Floortime. In 2015, Interplay Learning Academy was born with six students and six sets of parents that took a risk and trusted me with their child's education. It quickly grew and about a year after opening the doors, we moved to a new location that would allow us to accept more students with autism and other sensory motor differences.

At the beginning of 2016 Shelley reached out to me and said, "Dana, you *have* to see this!" She shared a video with me of one of her students spelling words on a stencil board after the teacher read a short passage of information. I was completely taken aback. How? I had read reports from psychologists and teachers talking about cognitive and intellectual delays in students with autism. In fact, the DSM-IV includes intellectual delay as part of the autism diagnosis so what was happening here? Shelley told me to look up RPM or Rapid Prompting Method and of course, I did right away. I needed to learn for myself what this was all about.

Soma M., a tiny Indian woman, taught her son Tito this method to demonstrate to the world that even though he couldn't communicate verbally, he was smart and had the ability to learn. Then it hit me. I recognized this woman from a *60 Minutes* episode I watched in 2003. I remember it vividly and thought how amazing it is that this woman has taught these kids to communicate. But how? I had so many questions and as I began to research and read articles, I became more and more discouraged. There was no research on this method. In fact, most if not all of the content that came up after a Google search suggested that this method was anything but miraculous and in fact could cause trauma. I was so confused. Why would Shelley suggest this? I had to learn more. So, I traveled back up north to see it for myself and to have a serious conversation with Shelley about my concerns.

I arrived at The Hirsch Academy soon after talking with Shelley over the phone and I remember sitting in the back of the classroom watching a student spell right in front of me. I couldn't "unsee" what I saw. This was amazing! Shelley then started talking about how students who are nonspeaking still have the ability to learn and just because they can't speak, doesn't mean that they don't understand. They just don't have the ability to demonstrate their knowledge and understanding. That was Soma's goal all along—to have her son demonstrate his knowledge. From that point on, everything changed for me. I went back and began reading books and blogs written by spellers and typers.

It hit me a short time after I left The Hirsch Academy, that I had been doing everything wrong. My students had the ability to learn and have been learning all along! They needed to have age-appropriate academic content. My clients needed more than just sensory integration. They needed to build their intentional motor skills. What the "issue" was wasn't an intellectual or cognitive issue, it was a motor issue—apraxia. This all made sense to me and it hit me hard. I thought of all the clients over the years who I had misunderstood and underestimated. They too struggled with the disconnect between their brain and body. They could all understand, but couldn't respond. Wow! My paradigm shift happened quickly, almost instantaneously actually.

I immediately changed the curriculum at school to be age-appropriate content. Yes, the teachers looked at me like I was crazy but at that point, I told them that they had to get on board the train or get off! One did get off but the rest took a leap of faith and stuck with me. We immediately saw changes in our students. They carried themselves with more confidence, they were more regulated during the day, and they seemed to soak it all in. It was unbelievable at times but over and over the staff talked about how this is life-changing for not only the students but for them as well.

My clinic also went through significant changes. Ido Kedar taught me that OT, from his experience, did nothing to help build the connection between his brain and body. It was when his mother hired a trainer that things for him started to change. That is what made the most difference for him because apraxia is the real issue. I immediately purchased a treadmill, weights, and other equipment so that I could support my clients the way that they needed to be supported. I learned nothing about this in my years of academia. It was always about autism as a cognitive or intellectual disability. We couldn't have been more wrong. It was my clients who really taught me what I needed to know and I will be forever grateful to them!

Now I am the founder of Spellers Center Tampa with a team of OTs and practitioners that are second to none. We meet families that are local and families that travel in to see us. Our areas of expertise include spelling and typing as communication but also supporting spellers to build intentional movement. Each day I feel blessed to be able to do what I do and work with families whose lives will be changed because their son or daughter now has a way to communicate.

Index

fluent, 153
frontal lobe, 83, 148, 154

G
gaze, 31, 43
gestural prompts, 68, 126, 154
Gore, Abigail, 143
grasping reflex, 85
gross motor, 14, 54, 58, 61–62, 69,
    85, 101, 148, 154
guilt, 26, 129

H
hand-eye coordination, 13,
    43, 65
Handley, Jamie, 33, 72
Handley, J.B., 28, 72
Hawking, Stephen, 7–8

I
ID. *See* intellectual disability (ID)
idea, 52
identity-first language, 10–11
IEP. *See* individualized education
    plan (IEP)
impulsivity, 48, 85–86, 89, 93–94
individualized education plan
    (IEP), 19, 60, 154
inhibit, 52, 104
initiating, 52, 99–100, 104,
    126–127
initiation prompts, 67, 126, 154
injurious behavior, 31–32, 47,
    89, 116
intake packet, 39, 47–48
intellectual disability (ID),
    14–15, 54

intentional movement, 9, 29–30,
    38, 42–45, 51–54, 67, 83–86,
    93–94, 97–98, 101, 104–105,
    121, 148–150, 155
interoception, 89, 111, 155

J
Jorgensen, Cheryl, 58–59

K
Kedar, Ido, 103
Keefer, Austin, 143–144
kinesthetic seeking, 92–93
King, Martin Luther, Jr., 27–28

L
language, speech *vs.*, 43–44,
    55–58
large 26, 63
least dangerous assumption, 25,
    28, 55, 58–59, 106, 119, 156

M
mathematics, 75–76
Maynard, Jack, 144
minimal speaker, 1–2, 11, 57, 156
Moro reflex, 85
motor coaching, 99–100, 130–131
motor continuum, 71–72
motor cortex, 12, 57, 83, 156
motor loops, 101–105, 156
motor planning, 42, 53–54
motor planning differences, 54
motor skills
    in acquisition phase, 81
    acquisition phase and, 147
    assessment and, 14–15